KU-004-047

Everyday English for International Nurses
A guide to working in the UK

Joy Parkinson BA
Author and Lecturer, London, UK

Chris Brooker BSc, MSc, RGN, SCM, RNT
Author and Lecturer, Norfolk, UK

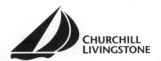

CHURCHILL LIVINGSTONE

EDINBURGH LONDON NEW YORK OXFORD PHILADELPHIA ST LOUIS
SYDNEY TORONTO 2004

CHURCHILL LIVINGSTONE
An imprint of Elsevier Limited

© 2004, Elsevier Limited. All rights reserved.

The right of Joy Parkinson and Chris Brooker to be identified as authors of this work has
been asserted by them in accordance with the Copyright, Designs and Patents Act 1988

No part of this publication may be reproduced, stored in a retrieval system, or transmitted in
any form or by any means, electronic, mechanical, photocopying, recording or otherwise,
without either the prior permission of the publishers or a licence permitting restricted
copying in the United Kingdom issued by the Copyright Licensing Agency, 90 Tottenham
Court Road, London W1T 4LP. Permissions may be sought directly from Elsevier's Health
Sciences Rights Department in Philadelphia, USA: phone: (+1) 215 238 7869, fax: (+1) 215
238 2239, e-mail: healthpermissions@elsevier.com. You may also complete your request online via the Elsevier homepage (http://www.elsevier.com), by selecting 'Customer Support'
and then 'Obtaining Permissions'.

First published 2004
    Reprinted 2006

ISBN 0 443 07399 6

British Library Cataloguing in Publication Data
A catalogue record for this book is available from the British Library

Library of Congress Cataloguing in Publication Data
A catalogue record for this book is available from the Library of Congress

Notice
Medical knowledge is constantly changing. As new information becomes available, changes
in treatment, procedures, equipment and the use of drugs become necessary. The editors,
contributor and the publishers have taken care to ensure that the information given in this
text is accurate and up to date. However, readers are strongly advised to confirm that the
information, especially with regard to drug usage, complies with the latest legislation and
standards of practice.

ELSEVIER your source for books,
journals and multimedia
in the health sciences
www.elsevierhealth.com

Working together to grow
libraries in developing countries

www.elsevier.com | www.bookaid.org | www.sabre.org

ELSEVIER   BOOK AID   Sabre Foundation
            International

The
publisher's
policy is to use
paper manufactured
from sustainable forests

Printed in China

610.73/PAR

Everyday English for International Nurses
A guide to working in the UK

KERRY GENERAL HOSPITAL LIBRARY

This book is due for return on or before the last date shown below.

For Churchill Livingstone:

Commissioning Editor: Ninette Premdas
Development Editor: Kim Benson
Project Manager: Darren Smith
Design: Erik Bigland

Preface

P/O NO:
ACCESSION NO. KHO1259
SHELFMARK: 610.73/PAR

This book is designed to help the large numbers of overseas nurses who have chosen to practise in the UK. The content has been adapted from the *Manual of English for the Overseas Doctor*, by Joy Parkinson. The result is a book with a uniquely nursing focus.

It can be a daunting prospect for anyone to move to another country to nurse; not only must you become familiar with the organisation and regulation of nursing, but you need to learn how English is spoken by people in everyday situations. The language spoken by clients, patients and their families in the UK is vastly different from that used overseas. Hence a large part of the book is concerned with the vocabulary and language used in the nurse–patient relationship.

The first three chapters provide information about nursing in the UK, the nursing process, professional organisations and trade unions, registering as a nurse, adaptation programmes and career development, and the structure of the National Health Service and Social Services.

Chapter 4 focuses on documentation and record keeping that are vital to good practice. This chapter also deals with written communication in the form of letters and e-mail.

Communication in nursing is covered in Chapter 5. This includes taking a nursing history and many case-history dialogues. The case histories are based on the Activities of Living Model of Nursing and provide examples of dialogue between nurses and patients or relatives in a wide range of situations.

Chapters 6 to 8 deal with the language of spoken English (colloquial English, idioms and phrasal verbs). This material is based on the book for doctors, but it has been completely updated for the 21st century.

The last three chapters provide you with more useful information – abbreviations used in nursing, useful addresses and web sources, and units of measurement.

Further reading suggestions and references are included in the chapters, and a general list of further reading is provided at the end of the book.

We hope that this new book will be of great help to you during your nursing career in the UK.

Joy Parkinson and Chris Brooker   London and Norfolk 2004

Acknowledgements

The authors would like to thank their families and colleagues for their support and help.

Thanks to Gosia Brykczynska who wrote the first three chapters.

Thanks also to Annie Jennings, RGN, and Andrew Jennings, MB, FRCS(Urol), for their help in updating the colloquial language, to Kirsten and Stuart Dallas who offered help with one of the case histories, and to all the staff at Elsevier who were involved in the book – in particular, Ninette Premdas and Kim Benson for their support and enthusiasm throughout the project.

Contributor

Gosia Brykczynska PhD, RGN/RSCN, RNT, CertEd, Refugee Nurse Project Officer, Royal College of Nursing, London, UK (Chs 1, 2 and 3).

Contents

Contents

Nursing in the UK

INTRODUCTION

Today nursing in the UK involves caring for the whole person (holistic care). This includes emotional, social, psychological, spiritual and physical factors rather than just a disease or injury. Nursing care is based on the best evidence available (evidence-based) and focuses on the individual needs of people using the healthcare system. Nurses are concerned as much with helping people to stay well, as with giving care when illness or injury occurs. Promoting health, giving information and helping people to learn about managing chronic illnesses is the focus of nursing in the 21st century. The developments in medical science and technology, and the breakdown in the traditional barriers between the healthcare professions have meant that nurses must now deal with many complex technical aspects of care and treatment. Nursing in the UK is a regulated professional occupation with a correspondingly thorough education system that meets the practical and theoretical needs of a modern healthcare system. Nurse education in the UK is designed to meet changing healthcare needs, the wishes of people needing healthcare, the growth in complex treatments and the need for a standardised educational preparation resulting from membership of the European Union (EU) (see Ch. 2).

Nurses in the UK base their practice on the systematic assessment, planning, implementation and evaluation of care. In order to do this they use the nursing process (see below) or integrated care pathways. This is very different to task-based care, where nursing activities were strictly allocated according to the nurse's seniority. The more complicated tasks, such as giving medicines, were performed by senior nurses and simple tasks were undertaken by the more junior nurses, while the most basic work such as personal cleansing was carried out by unqualified nursing students and nursing assistants or auxiliary nurses.

This chapter will help you to understand how nursing in the UK is regulated, what nurses do and where they work, and how they use the nursing process. Details about various professional organisations and trade unions are also given.

HOW NURSING IS REGULATED IN THE UK

Nursing and midwifery are regulated by the Nursing and Midwifery Council (NMC). The role of the NMC includes:

— Keeping a register of practitioners (656 000 qualified registered nurses and midwives in 2003). In 2004 a new three-part register – nursing, midwifery and specialist community public health nursing – replaced a register with 15 parts. The nursing part of the register has separate sections for first-level and second-level nurses. The register also notes the particular branch of nursing – adult, learning disability, children or mental health. The second-level section of the register is for existing enrolled nurses, but this is closed to new UK applicants. However, it must be open to existing second-level nurses who qualified in certain other European countries in order to comply with European Directives. All working nurses need to register with the NMC to practise as qualified nurses in the UK. This registration is renewed every 3 years (see periodic registration, Ch. 2).
— Setting standards for nursing and midwifery practice.
— Protecting the public and assuring the public that only nurses and midwives who have reached the minimum standards set by the NMC can become registered nurses and midwives.

The NMC hears cases of alleged professional misconduct (see nursing documentation and record keeping, Ch. 4). If the practitioner is found guilty, the NMC can deal with him or her in a variety of ways, including the removal of the practitioner from the professional register, which stops him or her working as a registered nurse or midwife. In this way, the NMC monitors and regulates nursing and midwifery and ensures that high standards of professional practice are maintained.

The NMC has produced a Code of Professional Conduct that sets out the standards of professional conduct, responsibilities and accountability expected of a registered nurse or midwife, and explains a person's entitlements and reasonable healthcare expectations about nursing care.

As part of the need to practise safely and effectively as a nurse and to work within ethical boundaries you need to be familiar with, to understand and to apply to your practice all parts of the Code of Professional Conduct. The main clauses of the code are outlined in Box 1.1, but you should read the full document which has subclauses that give more explanation.

The Code is sent to every practising nurse in the UK, and any nurse who does not respect the Code of Professional Conduct will have to answer for their actions or omissions to the NMC and others, including the hospital or care home where they work, a court of law or the Health Service Commissioner. The British public demand nursing care that is of a high standard and effective,

---

Box 1.1   The Code of Professional Conduct (NMC, 2002)

The Code of Professional Conduct says that, 'as a registered nurse or midwife, you are personally accountable for your practice. In caring for patients and clients, you must':

— 'respect the patient or client as an individual'
— 'obtain consent before you give any treatment or care' (see Ch. 4)
— 'co-operate with others in the team'
— 'protect confidential information'
— 'maintain your professional knowledge and competence'
— 'be trustworthy'
— 'act to identify and minimise the risk to patients and clients'.

Available online: http://www.nmc-uk.org

and nurses are constantly trying to raise their standards of care and to identify areas for improvement. In fact, continuing professional development (CPD) and a commitment to life-long learning are both essential if the profession is to keep ahead of the changes that are occurring and for nurses to feel confident in the work that they are doing. For more information about CPD, post-registration education and practice (PREP) and periodic registration, see Chapter 2.

PROFESSIONAL ORGANISATIONS AND TRADE UNIONS

The vast majority of practising UK nurses and midwives, and students join a professional organisation or trade union. There are several trade unions to choose from (Box 1.2), but the two most popular ones with nurses are the Royal College of Nursing (RCN) and Unison, who have about 600 000 members between them.

A trade union works hard for the welfare and best interests of its nurse members. Trade unions also provide professional indemnity insurance for practising nurse members, as do several private insurance companies. Nurses who are employed are covered for acts or omissions by their employer's vicarious liability arrangements. Professional indemnity insurance against claims for professional negligence is increasingly important for nurses work-

---

Box 1.2   Trade unions and professional organisations

— The Royal College of Nursing
— Unison
— The Royal College of Midwives (RCM)
— GMB
— Mental Health Nurses' Association
— Community Practitioners' and Health Visitors' Association
— Community and District Nurses' Association.

See Chapter 10 for useful addresses and websites.

ing in independent or private practice, and the NMC recommends that these nurses should have adequate insurance.

Many trade unions provide continuing education for nurses through study days, courses, conferences and nursing journals. Some organisations, notably the RCN and RCM, provide extensive libraries. Furthermore, the RCN has one of the largest non-university affiliated nursing libraries in the world.

The National Nursing Association (NNA) in the UK is the RCN. It is a member of the International Council of Nurses (ICN), and is the UK representative on the Standing Committee of Nurses in Europe.

More information about the services offered by individual trade unions and professional organisations can be found in an article by Oxtoby & Crouch (2003) and by contacting the trade union or professional organisation.

WHERE NURSES WORK – NATIONAL HEALTH SERVICE AND THE PRIVATE SECTOR

Most nurses and midwives (approximately 400 000) work for the National Health Service (NHS), 80 000 work in the private sector within independent hospitals, nursing homes, nursing agencies, workplaces, prisons, embassies and the armed forces, and 20 000 work for general practitioners (GPs). Others work in education institutions, in management, as independent practitioners, or as self-employed consultants.

In the 1980s, new nurse education programmes, called Project 2000 (PK2), were introduced. This moved nurse education into the higher education sector and nursing students were no longer considered part of the nursing workforce, as they had been before, and led to an increased employment of healthcare assistants (HCAs) and auxiliaries. HCAs often give the 'hands-on' care, and increasingly do more complex activities because the role of nurses has expanded and changed.

Nurses today work not only in hospitals but also in the community. In fact over a third of all UK nurses work in the community – with people in their own homes and in clinics, and in the workplace as occupational health nurses. Even when nurses are employed in the acute healthcare sector they not only work on the wards, but they also work in outpatient departments (OPDs) often running and co-ordinating clinics on their own, such as in pre-admission assessment, diabetic care, hypertension clinics, well-men and well-women clinics, and so on. In addition, UK nurses are increasingly taking on roles that used to be done by doctors. This has meant that nurses can now ensure a faster and more efficient service for people in their care.

Nurses in the UK can choose to work either for the NHS or for the private healthcare sector. The private sector runs hospitals (general and specialist), and many psychiatric hospitals and specialist clinics (e.g. infertility clinics and drug detoxification units). The private sector also provides much of the occupational health services for industry and many private companies, and run hundreds of nursing homes and other care facilities for older people and other groups all over the UK. The care of older people requires much dedication and is a difficult field of nursing, but it can be very rewarding and certainly it is an area of nursing care that will increase in demand as more people live longer, and proportionally more frail older people will require expert nursing care.

Although private healthcare establishments are not bound by NHS pay regulations, they generally pay very similar salaries and in many instances pay slightly more. There are recruitment guidelines and UK labour legislation helps to ensure fair and ethical employment practices. Wherever a nurse works in the UK he or she is protected by employment law and health and safety regulations which, among other things, specify the maximum number of hours of work to be undertaken in a specified period of time, the minimum UK wage, and employment entitlements and benefits.

Nursing in the UK reflects the challenges and the demands of UK society as a whole. Nursing is considered a respected and valued profession, and on the whole qualified nurses with several years' clinical experience and working full-time in a UK health-care establishment, can expect to be adequately financially rewarded for their expertise and practice. At the time of writing the government is proposing a new financial package for qualified nurses working in the NHS, which should redress some of the financial problems and dissatisfactions of the past.

HIGH QUALITY CARE AND THE NURSING PROCESS

Whether you are at the beginning of your career, practising at an advanced or specialist level, or just newly arrived to work in the UK from abroad, all nurses must strive to achieve the five Cs of good nursing practice:

— *competent* nursing
— *commitment* to nursing
— *confidence* in nursing research
— nursing *compassion*
— informed nursing *conscience*.

These aspects of caring nursing practice were first expressed by Simone Roach, a Canadian nurse, in 1984 (Roach 1984). All five aspects of nursing practice are needed for effective, high-quality nursing care. It is the caring aspect of nursing work that is most appreciated by people and their families, and nurses everywhere are delivering good patient care by demonstrating competency, commitment, confidence, conscience and compassion in their work. In many parts of the world, including the UK, these aspects of nursing care are best shown in nursing practice by using the nursing process.

The nursing process is a systematic approach to nursing care. It has four phases (Fig. 1.1):

— assessment
— planning
— implementation
— evaluation.

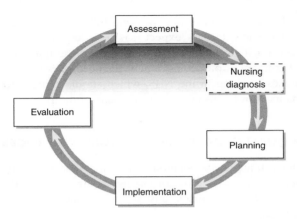

Fig. 1.1 The nursing process. Reproduced with permission from Brooker & Nicol (eds), *Nursing Adults: the Practice of Caring*, Mosby, 2003.

Although the four phases are described in sequence, in reality they overlap, and occur and recur throughout the period for which a person is receiving nursing care.

The nursing assessment refers to assessing a person (patient or client) for physical, psychological, social or spiritual needs and deciding on their relative nursing value. The status of the person is assessed in order to help with planning the nursing care plan.

The care plan is prepared with a specific person in mind; however, it is possible to have a prepared standard care plan, which is then adapted and individualised for a particular person's needs. This often happens on day-case surgery units and surgical wards where routine surgical procedures are undertaken. Such an approach ensures that not only are routine procedures undertaken, but also that the care can be individualised. Care plans may be hand written or, as is increasingly the case, stored on computers. In both instances, the information is confidential and should be held/stored in a safe place (see Ch. 4). In the UK, patients are entitled to know their diagnosis, to be included in care planning and to be consulted at every point of the nursing process cycle. This is to ensure fully informed and freely given consent to the care proposed (see Ch. 4).

The implementation of the care plan is based on the initial assessment process and the care delivered is expected to be evidence-based (i.e. in accordance with the latest nursing research findings and medical knowledge). If research findings are not available the evidence may be developed from the collection of best expert practice in the field. It is the responsibility of individual nurses to keep themselves updated in nursing practice, as they are individually accountable for patient care.

The final stage of the nursing process is the evaluation. At this point the nurse evaluates the effectiveness of the care delivered and either decides to continue with the current care plan, considers making changes, or moves on to another new assessment and care plan, as the person is now at another stage and has different needs. Evaluation must be undertaken against some measurement or established criteria (e.g. a pressure ulcer risk scale). This stage of the care plan is very important, as otherwise the nurse runs the risk of continuing to give ineffective and or inappropriate care.

The nursing process is used effectively by all nurses in the UK, regardless of their speciality, and as you gain clinical experience so it becomes easier to move through the stages of the process. As you would expect the nursing process needs a caring and knowledgeable approach and is usually made easier by using an established model or theory of nursing practice, such as the Roper, Tierney & Logan (1996) model of nursing based on activities of living or Orem's self-care model (1995). The result is that nursing care is being delivered more appropriately, effectively and in ways that promote holistic well-being.

Nurses should record all the relevant information at all stages of the nursing process (see Ch. 4).

AN EXCITING FUTURE – EXPANDING THE ROLE OF NURSES

In 1999 the UK Government issued a document for nurses to consider: NHS Plan for England (Department of Health 1999) in which it set out areas that it felt needed to be expanded and to become more mainstream, so that more nurses could be involved working in these areas in new and more challenging nursing roles. The areas were:

— to be capable of and responsible for ordering medical investigations, such as pathology tests and X-rays
— to be capable of making direct referrals to specialist services, such as a pain control team or the continence adviser
— to have responsibility for both admitting and discharging a range of patients with specified conditions according to a protocol
— for more nurses to manage their own patient caseloads, e.g. in the care of people with diabetes
— to increase the number of nurses who would be educated to prescribe medicines and treatments
— for nurses to be responsible for resuscitation procedures, including the use of defibrillation
— to be trained to undertake minor surgery and outpatient procedures
— to be responsible for the administration of outpatient clinics
— to take lead roles and executive positions in local health services and their management.

Nurses now have the chance to expand their practice, such as prescribing medicines, and diagnosing and treating many minor injuries and illnesses, as well as continuing to give holistic care, especially for those people with chronic conditions. Nurses work in ever more sophisticated and technologically advanced settings (e.g. in oncology units, endoscopy suites, neonatal units and renal and dialysis units). This requires a high level of basic nursing care, continuing post-basic specialist knowledge, a system of advanced nursing education to reflect the increased and variable nursing work environments and an ethical viewpoint that is informed and sensitive to the needs of people and their families. The next two chapters will help you to understand the routes and methods of achieving these specialisations and to have a basic understanding of the UK healthcare system and the role and function of nursing within it.

REFERENCES

Department of Health (DoH) 2000 The NHS plan. DoH, London.

Nursing and Midwifery Council (NMC) 2002 Code of professional conduct. NMC, London.

Orem DE 1995 Nursing: concepts and practice, 5th edn. Mosby, St. Louis.

Roach S 1984 Caring: the human mode of being, implications for nursing. Perspective in caring. Monograph 1. Faculty of Nursing, University of Toronto, Toronto.

Roper N, Logan WW, Tierney AJ 1996 The elements of nursing, 4th edn. Churchill Livingstone, Edinburgh.

FURTHER READING

Brooker C, Nicol M (eds) 2003 Nursing adults: the practice of caring. Mosby, Edinburgh, Ch. 1.

Oxtoby K, Crouch D 2003 Value for money. Nursing Times 99(17):21–23.

Royal College of Nursing (RCN) 2002 Labour market review. RCN, London.

Registering as a nurse in the UK and career development

INTRODUCTION

Of all the European countries, the UK has the largest number of overseas trained nurses working within the healthcare system. It is estimated that there are about 42 000 internationally recruited nurses practising in the UK, with another 16 000 waiting for placements on supervised practice courses. Every nurse who works in the UK needs to be registered with the Nursing and Midwifery Council (NMC). Since 1919 nurses have been regulated in the UK (Nurse Registration Act) and the NMC is the latest statutory body set up by Parliament to perform this regulatory role. The NMC was established in April 2002 and replaced The UK Central Council for Nursing, Midwifery and Health Visiting (UKCC). The change in regulatory body coincided with a change in the way that the nursing profession was to be organised and administered around the country and was in keeping with major changes occurring in the delivery of healthcare in the UK (see Ch. 3). One of the NMC's main functions is to protect the public by ensuring that all those who are registered to work as Registered Nurses (RNs) in the UK are considered to be safe and competent nursing practitioners (see Ch. 1).

This chapter will help you to understand how to obtain initial registration with the NMC and the requirements for periodic registration. There is further information about adaptation courses, and in addition the chapter will help you to develop your career and be successful as a nurse in the UK.

NURSING PROGRAMMES AND OBTAINING REGISTRATION

The first thing an overseas trained nurse must do to get onto the NMC register is to write to the NMC (for the address see Ch. 10) for an application pack. The pack gives information about payments and how to fill out the forms and what is needed to become a nurse in the UK. Information on how to apply to the NMC for registration can also be obtained from the NMC website (http://www.nmc-uk.org). The first sum of money you send off to the NMC is to cover the administration cost of processing the application forms. Refugee nurses do not have to pay the initial fee if they send the NMC a copy of the letter from the Home Office confirming their refugee status.

It is the NMC who will determine whether you are a safe and competent practitioner to work in the UK. This is done by looking at all applications on an individual basis. The NMC will assess several different things about you; for example, your nursing education, character references (from your school of nursing and employers), and experience and career pathway.

Nursing education models vary considerably around the world and Registered Nurses may undertake courses that last anything from 1 to 4 years. Some nurses have been educated at universities and colleges of higher education, others on pre-matriculation courses (before leaving secondary school) and also in specialised nursing further education institutes, which are often attached to specific teaching hospitals.

In some countries nursing programmes follow a universal healthcare career structure, where all or many of the healthcare workers progress together through a generic health worker training programme. However, some individuals remain at particular levels, while others will continue their education to gain more experience and thereby change the role that they are qualified to undertake. In other countries nurse education is completely separate from other healthcare professions. In the UK all nurse education, wherever it is provided, follows the European Union (EU) Directives on the nature and length of nurse education programmes.

The majority of overseas trained nurses will be seeking to have their name put on the nursing part of the register (for more information on the three-part register, see Ch. 1) and most of these will be for adult nursing. To be placed on the register you need to demonstrate that your nursing education programme meets the conditions outlined in Box 2.1.

These rules and regulations were agreed by the EU and have been agreed as valid for the whole of Europe. This was agreed in

---

Box 2.1   Nurse education programmes – conditions required for UK registration

— Duration of at least 3 years of full-time nursing studies and which included at least 4600 hours of nursing education. This means that unrelated subjects, such as foreign languages, sport or philosophy, do not count towards the nursing education hours, but applied subjects such as healthcare ethics would be relevant.

— The nursing programme does not have to be delivered at a degree level, but it should be undertaken after completion of full secondary education and after reaching the age of 17.

— The nursing programme needs to be equally divided between theory and practice and the programme must cover five main areas, i.e. medical, surgical, women and children, mental health and community.

— Upon completion of the nursing education programme, nursing students should be considered to be fully qualified registerable first-level nurses and fully capable of obtaining the nursing diploma and right to practise. This implies that the nursing education programme is considered to be complete in itself and without additional practice periods and/or supervision, and that until nursing students obtain the nursing diploma they are not considered to be fully qualified first-level nurses.

Apart from these requirements, the NMC requests that nurses complete at least 6 months of nursing work in their home country to consolidate their educational experience. Nurses trying to obtain UK registration without 6 months' experience in their home country might experience problems getting onto the register.

---

an effort to standardise the level of nurse education in Europe, and thereby enable automatic recognition of qualifications between the countries of the EU. Thus, if a qualified nurse from, for example, Zambia obtains nursing recognition from the NMC as a fully qualified first-level nurse in the UK, and obtains an NMC Professional Identification Number (PIN) and is put on the UK nursing register, the UK registration and recognition is valid throughout the whole of Europe. It means that Registered Nurses can easily move around within the EU for purposes of continuing nurse training and obtaining professional work.

The same rules ensure that the levels of nurse education are automatically raised overall. With the introduction of this type of nurse education the countries of Europe were asked to close their second-level nursing programmes. The only way to become a nurse in the EU today is by undertaking a 3-year programme of full-time education at post-secondary school level, as already described. The only nurses in Europe who are practising on the second-level register are those nurses who completed their training before the new regulations came into force, either from the UK or from other EU countries.

Will your application be accepted?

The NMC may accept your qualifications, require you to do an adaptation course, or insist on further training:

1. The NMC may fully recognise your qualifications, and because the education programme was conducted in English and it covered the European nursing education requirements you can be admitted onto the register without any additional requirements. This is the common situation if you have completed university degrees in nursing from North America, Australia or New Zealand and have sufficient additional practical nursing experience.
2. The vast majority of all other nurses will receive a letter from the NMC stating that their qualifications are sufficient for them to be put on the NMC register but that now they must com-

plete an adaptation programme (supervised practice) in an approved healthcare establishment in the UK over a specified period of time. This can range from 3 months to 1 year, but most commonly is for a period between 3 and 6 months.

3. Some non-EU trained nurses will be asked to undertake more pre-registration nurse education before they can be put on the UK register. Meanwhile, some of their original nurse training can be considered valid and academic credits can be awarded towards the new UK pre-registration nursing education. This process of giving credit for prior education is called Accreditation of Prior Experience and Learning (APEL). Every school of nursing in the UK can undertake this accreditation process for overseas-trained nurses. APEL was put into place to help adult mature entrants return to formal education to obtain new skills, and now this process is being extended to include previous achievements, even those gained overseas. It is a long process, but well worth undertaking.

The NMC may ask you for more information before they make a decision, or reject your application if your nursing course was less than 3 years long or you cannot meet other requirements (see Box 2.1).

Once you have completed all the requirements set by the NMC and sent your initial registration payment to the NMC, you will receive a PIN and a copy of the NMC Code of Professional Conduct (see Ch. 1).

Adaptation programmes (supervised practice)

Unfortunately there are not enough places on adaptation programmes. Although almost all acute NHS Trusts and many Primary Care Trusts (PCTs) do provide adaptation programmes, there are still not enough to provide adaptation placements for the large numbers of overseas trained nurses wishing to work in the UK.

Adaptation programmes for overseas trained nurses are run jointly by the NHS Trusts who provide access to the clinical areas and the necessary mentors and schools of nursing, who provide the lecturers and teaching support. Some approved supervised placements can also be undertaken in the independent sector, predominantly in care homes for older people. There is a shortage of placements for supervised practice because there are not enough qualified nurses to undertake the training necessary to become mentors, and the clinical areas are already completely full of pre- and post-registration nursing students. The authorities who commission and fund adaptation programmes are trying to increase the number of placements. The NMC is also beginning to look at other ways of assessing nurses' readiness to practise in the UK, such as by passing an examination, which may or may not include a clinical component, but all these alternatives are still a long way away.

It is because of these logistical problems that the NMC recommends that overseas trained nurses do not arrive in the UK until they have a guaranteed place on an approved adaptation course, since at the time of writing there is an estimated 2- to 3-year backlog in getting onto an adaptation programme in the UK.

Communication in English – International English Language Testing System

Overseas trained nurses need to be able to demonstrate the use of the English language to a level that is good enough to communicate with colleagues and patients and to function safely in the clinical environment. The NMC currently requires that all overseas trained nurses who completed their training in a language other than English need to pass the International English Language Testing System (IELTS) examination. The IELTS is a specific English language test that is administered by the British Council in centres worldwide. The IELTS test required for nurses is the General Test, and this consists of several sections, such as comprehension and communication. All these sections need to be completed successfully with a minimum grade of 5.5; however, an overall grade of 6.5 must finally be achieved. Many nurses find the examination difficult and not necessarily appropriate for nursing practice. The NMC is considering several other possibilities, but one thing is sure – nurses whose first language is not English will need to demonstrate that they have a reasonable command of the English language. In addition to needing sufficient English to function safely in clinical areas and with patients, overseas trained nurses will need the equivalent of IELTS grade 6.5 in order to undertake further nursing education at a UK university.

PERIODIC REGISTRATION AND CONTINUING PROFESSIONAL DEVELOPMENT

Periodic registration

The nursing register is constantly being updated, and you will need to update your right to be on the register by periodic registration. The right to practise as a nurse in the UK is not only dependent on paying an initial fee, but you must also complete a Notification of Practice form every 3 years and pay another fee, and fulfil certain requirements for post-registration education and practice (PREP) (Box 2.2).

Continuing professional development

Continuing professional development (CPD) can be gained in a number of ways, for example:

— Reading professional articles in the nursing press, such as the *Professional Nurse*, *Nursing Times* or *Nursing Standard*. Doing literature searches relevant to your area of practice.
— Visiting other units.
— Ward teaching sessions, study days, conferences or seminars.
— Short courses, such as moving and handling, managing aggression and pain control. Longer courses, such as a degree, or studies that lead to registration on another part of the NMC nursing register, or the community public health nursing or midwifery parts of the register.

The important thing is that you are able to demonstrate an approach to professional nursing that is consistent with the principles of life-long learning. The way to do this is to keep a personal professional profile/portfolio that contains evidence of all the CPD activities you have achieved over a 3-year period. This is a requirement for PREP, and if you keep your profile up to date you will always be ready for periodic registration.

It is vital to reflect on your CPD activities, so you can identify what you have learned and its relevance to your practice. Reflection is an important part of all nursing activity, which of course ties into the evaluation stage of the nursing process (see Ch. 1). Many overseas trained nurses will already have been asked to undertake a reflective diary on their adaptation course, so you will probably be familiar with this approach. Reflecting on personal nursing practice is crucial to meaningful CPD.

Box 2.2   Post-registration education and practice (PREP)

The requirements for periodic registration are:

— undertake a minimum of 5 days or 35 hours of learning that is relevant to their practice (see Continuing Professional Development (CPD), p. 19)
— work in some capacity by virtue of their nursing qualifications for a minimum of 750 hours (100 days) during the last 5 years, or have done a return to practice course
— keep a personal professional profile of their learning (see Further Reading and Resources at the end of this chapter)
— comply with any request by the NMC to check (audit) how the requirements have been met.

The NMC states that the CPD requirements for PREP can be achieved in many different ways and need not cost a lot of money (see Further Reading and Resources at the end of this chapter).

DEVELOPING YOUR CAREER

Some adaptation placements, nursing courses and all job vacancies are published in the nursing press and sometimes in local newspapers. It may also be a good idea to go to the local hospital or PCT headquarters and look at the job vacancies bulletin board. The NMC also provides a website of job vacancies (http://www.nmc4jobs.com). Whether you are applying for an adaptation placement or for a first nursing job after completing the supervised practice, you will need to complete a curriculum vitae (CV) (see Further Reading and Resources at the end of this chapter), to fill out an application form, and if short-listed you will need to attend an interview. It is really important that the application form is filled out correctly and that your CV is complete, so that the reader (i.e. the prospective employer) knows who you are, what you have done and why you want the job. If you do not provide all the information you are unlikely to get short-listed for an interview.

Many teachers of English as a Second Language (ESOL) and IELTS classes will help you write a CV and explain how to fill out application forms. In addition, you can ask for help from Job Centres or your nursing mentors, whoever is more accessible and appropriate. There are also many books about how to complete application forms and a CV, and how to prepare for interviews. These can be found in public and nursing libraries.

Preparing for a job interview is time well spent – you should, for example, be familiar with the job description and any special responsibilities of the post (see Further Reading and Resources at the end of this chapter). If you are unable to attend on the date given for an interview it is considered polite to inform the personnel department; as they were impressed enough to invite you for interview they may well offer you another date. It is essential to give yourself plenty of time to get to the interview, to be punctual, to be prepared and to be positive about the experience, however nervous you may be. If you find you are going to be late for a reason beyond your control, it is a good idea if at all possible to telephone and explain the situation. That way, they may even offer you another time to attend the interview.

At the start of your UK nursing career (whether in the National Health Service (NHS) or the private sector) you will be placed on a fairly basic salary grade, most probably grade D or E (see Ch. 3). When you are ready for more responsibility and can work in more specialised areas you will be given the opportunity to apply for more senior posts and develop your nursing career. The NHS pay and career structure is undergoing change, and a new system of payment and assessing workloads and work definitions is being piloted and will then be introduced nationwide (*Agenda for Change*, Department of Health 1999).

Most employers require nurse managers, including ward sisters and charge nurses to have at least a first degree in nursing or a relevant subject and usually evidence of specialisation in the work undertaken in the clinical area. Nursing degrees (first and higher degrees) are offered by schools of nursing which are based in universities. A degree can last from between 1 and 3 years, depending on the existing level of nursing education. There are many opportunities for advancing your nursing career through education, and many of these are sponsored by the NHS.

It is common nowadays for your manager to do periodic reviews of your work with you. When you have a review meeting it is important to talk about your career plans and to start mapping out (planning and deciding) how you plan to achieve your nursing goals. Moving around clinical areas is one way of gaining new experience, but most UK nurses progress slowly through a given specialty, becoming more expert in specific aspects of nursing care (e.g. pain control, stoma care, tissue viability or substance misuse).

REFERENCES

Department of Health (DoH) 1999 Agenda for change. DoH, London.

FURTHER READING AND RESOURCES

Banks C 2003 How to ... excel at interview. Nursing Times 99(33):58–59.

Hyde J 2002 In: Brooker C (ed). Churchill Livingstone's dictionary of nursing, 18th edn. Churchill Livingstone, Edinburgh, p 512–518.

Hoban V 2003 How to ... write a CV. Nursing Times 99(27):52–53.

Registering as a nurse or midwife in the UK, see the NMC website: http://www.nmc-uk.org

The National Health Service and Social Services

INTRODUCTION

Since 1948 the healthcare system in the UK has been structured around the National Health Service (NHS) and social welfare has been delivered by local Social Service agencies. Both systems are maintained from the contributions of UK taxpayers, but the services are available to everyone, whether they pay taxes or not, such as children and some older people.

Although the NHS and Social Services have changed dramatically over the years, most people in the UK still want a national healthcare and social welfare system to continue to serve the whole population. Currently, the NHS is undergoing further structural change, which is aimed at improving the services to the public and making NHS workers more accountable to patients and UK taxpayers.

There are over a million people working for the NHS, as healthcare professionals and individuals supporting the clinical staff, such as electricians, gardeners, managers and clerical staff. The public sector NHS provides over 75% of the healthcare delivered in the UK.

This chapter will help you understand how the NHS is organised in England (services in Wales may be different and in Scotland services are organised differently) and explain the various roles of people within the NHS and the close links between the NHS and Social Services.

THE STRUCTURE OF THE NHS

The NHS is the responsibility of the Department of Health (DoH) with a remit to deliver comprehensive healthcare to the public. This ranges from primary care, including access to general practitioners (GPs), screening programmes, maternity care, mental health, secondary (surgical and medical) care in hospitals, specialist hospitals, and through to care of chronically ill people and those needing palliative care.

New developments in medical science place extra demands on the NHS and means that treatment provision needs to keep changing, as do the medicines that doctors and nurses can prescribe. It is one of the aims of the DoH to ensure that all treatments delivered by the NHS are evaluated and evidence based. The National Institute for Clinical Excellence (NICE) is the government agency set up to evaluate new treatments and drugs and provide guidance (see Further Reading and Resources at the end of this chapter). This is to guarantee that the best care is delivered by the most cost-effective method.

In the last few years the DoH has launched NHS Direct, an innovative service with a completely new approach to healthcare. NHS Direct is a telephone helpline (0845 4647), which aims to empower individuals and prevent the inappropriate use of GPs and emergency departments for minor conditions, by providing information and healthcare advice. NHS Direct is operated 24 hours a day by qualified nurses and health workers. The operators recommend what the caller should do (e.g. call an emergency ambulance, make an appointment to see their GP, or take a simple self-care remedy). The service empowers people to take responsibility for their health and the choices that they make. NHS Direct also provides web-based information about healthcare and the NHS (www.nhsdirect.nhs.uk).

The DoH manages the overall health and social care system, develops policy and manages changes in the NHS, regulates and inspects health and social care establishments and services and intervenes when necessary to improve services.

The work of the DoH is divided into two main areas:

— Strategic Health Authorities (SHAs), based on specific geographical regions. The SHAs ensure that NHS Trusts deliver the healthcare that has been commissioned, and they oversee various aspects of workforce planning (e.g. monitoring and arranging the training of healthcare workers, including nurses). They work with NHS Trusts and universities to plan and support clinical placements for overseas trained nurses (see Ch. 2). The SHA is responsible for strategic healthcare planning and for ensuring that national priorities are integrated into the work of the Primary Care Trusts (PCTs) and NHS Trusts (see below). Thus the SHA is concerned with primary healthcare and community services, which are organised by the PCTs, and acute hospital (secondary) services provided by NHS Trusts. Mental healthcare (delivered by mental health nurses) may be delivered either through the services of a special Psychiatric NHS Trust (covering inpatient and outpatient/community services) or by a Community NHS Trust (i.e. a PCT) or a General NHS Hospital Trust.

— Special health authorities, called Special Trusts. Special Trusts are usually considered to be secondary care providers or sometimes tertiary referral centres, such as the Hospital for Sick Children in London. Other Special Trusts include some inpatient units designated for forensic psychiatry.

Primary Care Trusts

PCTs work closely with Social Services (see below) and other agencies and organisations to assess local health needs, plan, develop and deliver community and primary healthcare services, and commission secondary services for the local population, in order to improve health and reduce inequalities in health. PCTs are responsible for public health and various intermediate care services. The SHA is responsible for the performance management of PCTs. Over recent years there has been a huge shift in how and where healthcare is delivered and much more care is provided within the community (person's home, care homes, NHS walk-in centres, healthcare clinics, etc.) by Primary Healthcare Teams (PHCTs) comprising nurses, midwives, doctors, therapists, etc. In addition, pharmacists, dentists, opticians and optometrists, and podiatrists all work within the community.

Primary Healthcare Team

GPs usually work in a group practice with several doctors who work within a team comprising practice nurses, district nurses (DNs), health visitors (HV), community midwives, community mental health nurses, physiotherapists, occupational therapists, speech and language therapists, counsellors and podiatrists, etc. Other professionals involved include school nurses (school health advisers), dieticians, etc. The PHCT delivers basic medical services, community care and liaises with local acute NHS Trusts for the continued and ongoing care of their patients. Practice nurses and GPs are usually the first point of contact for the person who is unwell or needs healthcare advice.

The nursing and midwifery roles within the team include:

— The practice nurse is a Registered Nurse (adult) who works alongside the GP in the GP surgery and often runs specialised clinics (e.g. immunisation, family planning and diabetic clinics). Some practice nurses are also nurse practitioners who perform many activities that are considered to be an extension of traditional nursing roles. Nurse practitioners are educated (usually to degree level) to diagnose and manage many basic conditions and to prescribe medications from the *Nurse Prescribers' Formulary* (NPF). Suitably qualified district nurses and health visitors also prescribe from the NPF.
— District nurses (DNs), who are also called community nurses, are responsible for the nursing care provided for people in their homes or in care homes. DNs are Registered Nurses (usually adult branch, although some are paediatric or learning disability nurses) who have undertaken additional education at a university to obtain a degree in community nursing. A DN usually supervises a small nursing team of staff nurses and

nursing assistants. Various health and social care professionals may ask for a DN to assess a person in their home or a patient may make a self-referral; similarly, a hospital may request that a DN provide nursing care for a person following discharge from hospital.

— Health visitors (HV) are Registered Nurses who have undergone further university nursing education in order to work in the community and who specialise in health promotion, health education and health maintenance. HVs do not deliver hands-on nursing care. They concentrate on the welfare of small children and mothers, but some HVs also work with older people or groups with specific needs, such as refugees. In every geographical area there will be a designated HV who is responsible for children with special needs and those children who may be at risk of being neglected or abused physically, mentally or sexually by their parents or carers.

— Community midwives provide professional care during pregnancy and labour and look after newly delivered mothers and their babies in the community. Most babies are born in a District General Hospital in the UK and in many areas community midwives accompany women into hospital to conduct the delivery and take the woman and new baby home after a few hours if all is well. Community midwives attend home births, especially for women who have already had a child and are expected to have a straightforward delivery. They also provide care for women who have been discharged following a booked hospital delivery. In an uncomplicated delivery the woman and baby are often discharged home to the care of the community midwife within 12 hours.

— Community mental health nurses also work in the community, but they specialise in the care of people with mental health problems. They work with people in their own homes, community-based mental health units, drugs and alcohol services and the criminal justice system. They liaise with other members of the PHCT, psychiatrists from local NHS Mental Health Trusts, clinical psychologists and social workers.

Other community health professionals
See Box 3.1 for an outline.

Ambulance Trusts

The Ambulance Service provides emergency care in the event of serious illness or accident. Ambulance paramedics will stabilise the person's condition and then transport them to the most appropriate emergency department (e.g. the local District General Hospital). There is no charge for an emergency ambulance, which is summoned by telephoning (999). You must ask the operator for an ambulance, explaining as clearly as possible the nature of the problem and the location. The Ambulance Service itself is divided into emergency services and patient transport services.

Secondary Care – NHS Acute Care Trusts

Secondary hospital care in the UK is delivered by NHS Trusts. Acute care hospitals and some inpatient continuing care units (e.g. for the care of older people) are part of NHS Trusts. Hospitals are managed by a chief executive who is accountable to the Executive Board of the Hospital Trust. Increasingly, the management of hospitals is delegated to specific clinical directorates within the Trust. Secondary care is provided in outpatient departments, day case units and inpatient beds.

Nursing staff
Many nurses wear a uniform of some sort, which varies from hospital to hospital and even within a hospital according to rank but also according to nursing department. For example, paediatric nurses often wear colourful tops and tabards, while those in intensive care wear theatre tops and trousers, and mental health nurses and senior nurses may wear their own clothes.

Within each Hospital Trust there will be a chief nurse (who may be known as the nursing director, etc), who also sits on the

---

Box 3.1   Other health professionals working in the community

— *Community pharmacists:* most work within the NHS although they are independent practitioners. A typical pharmacist on the high street will have a working relationship with their local GP surgeries. Medicines and surgical/nursing supplies written out on a GP's or nurse's prescription form will be dispensed by the pharmacist. A standard NHS prescription charge applies to each item, but most people are exempt and do not pay for prescriptions. These include children and pregnant women, people aged over 60 years, people receiving certain social security benefits and people with certain conditions (e.g. diabetes mellitus). Community pharmacists also offer advice to the public about minor ailments and all aspects of medication.

— *Dentists* are independent practitioners and some work with NHS patients and provide services to patients at NHS rates. However, there are few dentists who provide care under the NHS and currently PCTs are employing more dentists to deliver NHS dental care. There are several NHS dental hospitals in the UK, which provide for patients with maxillofacial and dental problems. These hospitals also train and provide practical placements for specialist personnel such as *dental nurses* and *speech and language therapists* and of course dentists and *postgraduate dental surgeons*.

— *Opticians* are also independent practitioners, but most work with NHS patients and provide services to people at NHS rates. Some *optometrists* and opticians work in NHS hospitals, but the majority practise in the community. Certain groups of people do not pay for eye care; these include pregnant women and children. People aged over 60 years and those with conditions such as diabetes or glaucoma are exempt from some charges.

Trust board. The chief nurse provides professional nursing leadership and is responsible for the overall implementation of nursing policies in a Trust and for the smooth running of the nursing department.

Currently the nursing posts open to qualified Registered Nurses are graded from D to I:

— A *D grade staff nurse* is considered the first nursing post that a newly qualified nurse undertakes. A D grade post is really a 'consolidation' post, where the new nurse graduate consolidates the training and education that he or she has received before seeking promotion after a year or two. Initially, most overseas trained nurses will be D grade until they become used to nursing in the UK. However, depending on a nurse's previous experience and learning, he or she may be upgraded very quickly.

— An *E grade* is for a *more experienced staff nurse.*

— A staff nurse is responsible to the *F or G grade* nurse known as the *ward sister/charge nurse (male) or ward manager.* Some hospitals use F grade for senior staff nurses, whereas others use it for junior ward sisters/charge nurses. Apart from staff nurses, ward sisters/charge nurses, healthcare assistants and nursing students there will be senior nurses, clinical nurse specialists, research nurses, lecturer–practitioners and nurse consultants who are also employed by some PCTs.

— *Senior nurses (G, H or I grade)* usually have a managerial role as well as responsibilities for a clinical speciality. Some senior nurses have responsibility for several wards or units and they are responsible to a general manager for organisational issues and to the chief nurse for professional issues. Some senior nurses have taken on the role of the modern 'matron', a post that is intended to give mid-level nursing managers more authority over hospital matters, and especially control over issues such as the cleanliness of the hospital. There are many clinical nurse specialists working in hospitals (and the community), especially in specialised areas such as pain control, palliative care, stoma care and oncology. The nurse will have undergone further education at a university and be a role model for colleagues, acting as mentor and educationalist. The lecturer–practitioner has a commitment to a student group at a university, teaches and undertakes nursing research, in addition to the role of specialist nurse.

There is quite a difference between the pay of the D grade nurse who is starting a career in nursing and a G or H grade nurse. However, this pay arrangement is in the process of change, as the government is piloting a new system of payment and assessing workloads and work definition (Department of Health 1999) prior to its introduction nationwide. The new pay deal will be beneficial to junior nurses, but to progress in the nursing career structure it is necessary to undertake further training and education (see Ch. 2).

Medical staff

Medical staff posts in hospitals are structured, with the post of consultant (e.g. a nephrologist) being at the top of the clinical speciality:

— Consultant: a physician or surgeon who has completed a lengthy postgraduate specialisation.
— Associate specialist: an experienced doctor who is nominally under the supervision of the consultant.
— Staff grade: a doctor who provides support for consultants.
— Specialist registrar: a doctor undertaking higher specialist training.
— Senior house officer: a doctor undertaking basic specialist training.
— House officer (pre-registration): a newly qualified doctor in the year following qualification.

Surgeons in the UK are addressed as Mr or Mrs/Miss/Ms.

The introduction of European Union Working Directives has reduced junior doctors' hours and this has meant that some nurses are trained to undertake some of the work traditionally done by junior doctors.

Professions allied to medicine and other staff

There are many other groups of professionals working in hospitals (e.g. radiographers, technicians, medical scientists, physiotherapists, speech and language therapists, play therapists, teachers (in children's hospitals) and social workers). You will also encounter translators and healthcare advocates, who are bilingual native speakers of various languages.

SOCIAL SERVICES

Social Services are provided by Local Authorities (local government). For example, Norfolk County Council provides services for the people who live in the county of Norfolk. Social Service departments have a statutory responsibility to provide care for groups that include:

— children and young people
— people with disabilities, including sensory impairments
— people who have problems with alcohol and drugs
— older people
— people with mental health problems.

Care and support is provided in the person's own home or in small community-based care units. People needing these services will have a named social worker to co-ordinate and monitor the care package. The care package may include help with personal care, day centres, respite care and home modifications such as bath rails and stair lifts.

As you advance in your UK nursing career you will have a great deal of contact with social workers. Joint working between health and social care professionals is vital for effective care planning and delivery. This is especially so in discharge planning, and in the community where there is considerable overlap between the work of health and social care professionals. In many areas, such as mental health and children, health and Social Services have formed a single Social Services & NHS Trust which aims to provide high-quality care.

REFERENCES

Department of Health (DoH) 1999 Agenda for change. DoH, London.

FURTHER READING AND RESOURCES

Clinical guidance, see the National Institute for Clinical Excellence (NICE) website: www.nice.org.uk

Medicines and healthcare products, see the Medicines and Healthcare products Regulatory Agency (MHRA) website: www.mhra.gov.uk

Public health (infection control, poisons, chemical and radiation hazards), see the Health Protection Agency (HPA) website: www.hpa.org.uk

Nursing documentation, record keeping and written communication

4

INTRODUCTION

Accurate record keeping and careful documentation is an essential part of nursing practice. The Nursing and Midwifery Council (NMC 2002) state that 'good record keeping helps to protect the welfare of patients and clients' – which of course is a fundamental aim for nurses everywhere. You can look at the full Guidelines for records and record keeping by visiting the NMC website (www.nmc-uk.org).

It is equally important that you can also communicate by letter and e-mail with other health and social care professionals, to ensure that they understand exactly what you mean.

NURSING DOCUMENTATION AND RECORD KEEPING

High quality record keeping will help you give skilled and safe care wherever you are working. Registered Nurses have a legal and professional duty of care (see Code of Professional Conduct, Ch. 1). According to the Nursing and Midwifery Council guidelines (NMC 2002) your record keeping and documentation should demonstrate:

— a full description of your assessment and the care planned and given
— relevant information about your patient or client at any given time and what you did in response to their needs
— that you have understood and fulfilled your duty of care, that you have taken all reasonable steps to care for the patient or

client and that any of your actions or things you failed to do have not compromised their safety in any way

— 'a record of any arrangement you have made for the continuing care of a patient or client'.

Investigations into complaints about care will look at and use the patient/client documents and records as evidence, so high quality record keeping is essential. The hospital or care home, the NMC, a court of law or the Health Service Commissioner may investigate the complaint, so it makes sense to get the records right. A court of law will tend to assume that if care has not been recorded then it has not been given.

Documentation

You will see lots of different charts, forms and documentation. Every hospital, care home and community nursing service will have the same basic ones, but with small variations that work best locally. The common documents that you will use include some of the following.

Nursing assessment sheet

The nursing assessment sheet contains the patient's biographical details (e.g. name and age), the reason for admission, the nursing needs and problems identified for the care plan, medication, allergies and medical history.

Nursing care plan

The documents of the care plan will have space for:

— Patient/client needs and problems.
— Sometimes, nursing diagnoses will be documented but these are not used as frequently as in North America.
— Planning to set care priorities and goals. Goal-setting should follow the SMART system, i.e. the goal will be specific, measurable, achievable and realistic, and time-oriented. For exam-

ple, a SMART goal would be that 'Mr Lee will be able to drink 1.5 L of fluid by 22.00 hours'. Some goals, such as reducing anxiety, are not easily measured and it is usual to ask patients to describe how they feel about a problem that was causing anxiety.

— The care/nursing interventions needed to achieve the goals.
— An evaluation of progress and the review date. This might include evaluation notes, continuation sheets and discharge plans. In some care areas you might record progress using a Kardex system along with the care plan.
— Reassessing patient/client needs and changing the care plan as needed.

Vital signs

The basic chart is used to record temperature, pulse, respiration and possibly blood pressure. Sometimes the patient's blood pressure is recorded on a separate chart. Basic charts may also have space to record urinalysis, weight, bowel action and the 24-hour totals for fluid intake and output. More complex charts, such as neurological observation charts, are used for recording vital signs plus other specific observations, which include the Glasgow Coma Scale score for level of consciousness, pupil size and reaction to light, and limb movement (Fig. 4.1).

Fluid balance chart

This is often called a 'fluid intake and output chart' or sometimes just 'fluid chart'. It is used to record all fluid intake and fluid output over a 24-hour period. The amounts may be totalled and the balance calculated at 24.00 hours (midnight), or at 06.00 or 08.00 hours. Sometimes the amounts are totalled twice in every 24 hours (i.e. every 12 hours). Fluid intake includes oral, nasogastric, via a gastrostomy feeding tube, and infusions given intravenously, subcutaneously and rectally. Fluid output from urine, vomit, aspirate from a nasogastric tube, diarrhoea, fluid from a stoma or wound drain are all recorded (Fig. 4.2).

OBSERVATION CHART

NAME:

HOSP. No.:

AGE:

CONSULTANT:

DATE:

TIME:

C O M A	Eyes open	Spontaneously	Eyes closed by swelling = C
		To speech	
		To pain	
		None	
S C A L E	Best verbal response	Orientated	Endotracheal tube or tracheostomy = T
		Confused	
		Inappropriate words	
		Incomprehensible sounds	
		None	
	Best motor response	Obey commands	Usually record the best arm response
		Localise pain	
		Flexion to pain	
		Extension pain	
		None	

Blood pressure and pulse rate

240
230
220
210
200
190
180
170
160
150

1 ·
2 •
3 ●
4 ⬤

Temperature °C
40
39
38
37
36
35
34
33
32

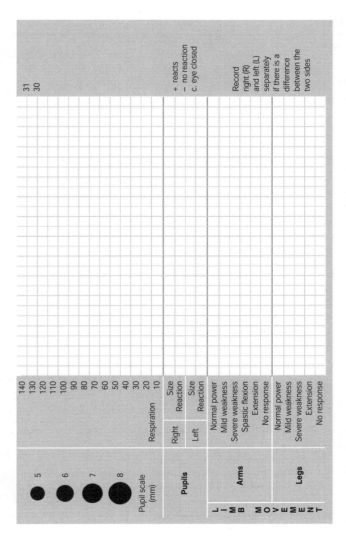

Fig. 4.1 Neurological observation chart: the Glasgow Coma Scale. Reproduced with permission from Brooker & Nicol (eds), *Nursing Adults: the Practice of Caring*, Mosby, 2003.

Fluid balance chart

Hospital/Ward:			Date:					
Hospital number:								
Surname:								
Forenames:								
Date of birth:								
Sex:								

	Fluid intake			Fluid output				
Time (hrs)	Oral	IV	Other (specify route)	Urine	Vomit	Other (specify)		
01.00								
02.00								
03.00								
04.00								
05.00								
06.00								
07.00								
08.00								
09.00								
10.00								
11.00								
12.00								
13.00								
14.00								
15.00								
16.00								
17.00								
18.00								
19.00								
20.00								
21.00								
22.00								
23.00								
24.00								
TOTAL								

Fig. 4.2   Fluid balance chart. Reproduced with permission from Nicol et al, *Essential Nursing Skills*, Mosby, 2000.

Medicine/drug chart

It is important for you to become familiar with the medicine/drug-related documents used in your area of practice. A basic medication record will contain the patient's biographical information, weight, history of allergies and previous adverse drug reactions. There will be separate areas on the chart for different types of drug orders. These include:

— drugs to be given once only at a specified time, such as a sedative before an invasive procedure
— drugs to be given immediately as a single dose and only once, such as adrenalin (epinephrine) in an emergency
— drugs to be given when required, such as laxatives or analgesics (pain killers)
— drugs given regularly, such as a 7-day course of an antibiotic or a drug taken for longer periods (e.g. a diuretic or a drug to prevent seizures).

All drugs, except a very few, are ordered using the British Approved Name, and the order (or prescription) will include the dose, route, frequency (with times), start date and sometimes a finish date. There is space for the signature of the nurse giving the drug and, in some cases, the witness. It is vital to record when you give a drug. This is done at the time so that all staff know that it has been given, and do not repeat the dose. Likewise, if you cannot give the drug for some reason (e.g. patient is in another department or their physical condition contraindicates giving the drug), make sure that this fact is recorded on the medicine/drug chart and the doctor is informed if necessary.

Remember that in some situations you will need to record in the nursing notes when you give patients a drug (e.g. if you give analgesic drugs (pain killers)).

Informed consent

Responsibility for making sure that the person or the parents of a child have all the information needed for them to give informed written consent rests with the health practitioner (usually a doctor or nurse) who is undertaking the procedure or operation. This information will include:

— information about the procedure/operation
— the benefits and likely results
— the risks of the procedure/operation
— the other treatments that could be used instead
— that the patient/parent can consult another health practitioner
— that the patient/parent can change their mind.

Young people can sign the consent form once they reach the age of 16 years and/or have the mental capacity to understand fully all that is involved. If the young person cannot sign the form, the parent or legal guardian may sign it. If an adult lacks the mental capacity, either temporarily or permanently, to give or deny consent, no person has the right to give approval for a course of action. However, treatment may be given if it is considered to be in the person's best interests, as long as an explicit (clear) refusal to such action has not been made by the person in advance.

Doctors do most invasive procedures and operations, but nurses in the UK are extending their practice to include many procedures that were previously done by doctors. You may work with nurses who do procedures such as endoscopic examinations, so it is becoming more common for nurses to obtain informed consent. The patient or parent and the healthcare practitioner both sign the consent form.

When your patients are due to have any invasive procedure, always check their level of understanding before it is scheduled to happen. If you are not sure about answering a question, ask the healthcare practitioner who is doing the procedure to see the patient and explain again. It is essential that the consent form is signed before the patient is given a sedative or other premedication drugs.

Incident/accident form

Any non-routine incident or accident involving a patient/client, relative, visitor or member of staff must be recorded by the nurse who witnesses (sees) the incident or finds the patient/client after the incident happened. Incidents include falls, drug errors, a visitor fainting or a patient attacking a member of staff in any way.

An incident/accident form should be completed as soon as possible after the event. Careful documentation of incidents is important for clinical governance (continuous quality improvement, learning from mistakes and managing risk, etc.) and in case of a complaint or legal action (see above).

The following points provide you with some guidance:

— be concise, accurate and objective
— record what you saw and describe the care you gave, who else was involved and the person's condition
— do not try to guess or explain what happened (e.g. you should record that side rails were not in place, but you should not write that this was the reason the patient fell out of bed)
— record the actions taken by other nurses and doctors at the time
— do not blame individuals in the report
— always record the full facts.

Guidelines for documentation and record keeping

The basic guidelines for good practice in documentation and record keeping apply equally to written records and to computer-held records.

The Nursing and Midwifery Council (NMC 2002) has said that patient and client records should:

— be based on fact, correct and consistent
— be written as soon as possible after an event has happened to provide current (up to date) information about the care and condition of the patient or client
— 'be written clearly and in such a way that the text cannot be erased' (rubbed out or obliterated)
— be written in such a way that any alterations or additions are dated, timed and signed, so that the original entry is still clear
— 'be accurately dated, timed and signed, with the signature

printed alongside the first entry' (this is even more important because your last name may not be very common in the UK)
— 'not include abbreviations, jargon, meaningless phrases, irrelevant speculation and offensive subjective statements'
— 'be readable on any photocopies'.

Note: Although the NMC guidelines clearly state that abbreviations should not be used in patient/client records, because you will see and hear abbreviations used in medical notes and handover reports, a list of commonly used ones is provided in Chapter 9 to help you understand what people mean.

The NMC goes on to say that records should:

— 'be written, wherever possible, with the involvement of the patient, client or their carer'
— 'be written in terms that the patient or client can understand'
— 'be consecutive' (uninterrupted)
— 'identify problems that have arisen and the action taken to rectify' (correct or put right) them
— 'provide clear evidence of the care planned, the decisions made, the care delivered and the information shared'.

OTHER WRITTEN COMMUNICATION

Letter writing

Letters may be professional, business or private. The private type is obviously easier to write, but there are, nevertheless, certain basic rules to be remembered.

The envelope

— It is becoming increasingly common in the UK to put the sender's name and address on the back of the envelope, particularly when sending packages and important documents. However, most people in the UK throw away envelopes as soon as letters are opened, so if you want an answer you must write your full address on the letter itself.
— It is correct to address people as Mr, Ms, Mrs or Miss with ini-

tials and last name (e.g. Miss J Smith or Mr O Massoud). Many women prefer to be addressed as Ms, regardless of marital status, and certainly Ms should be used where you are unsure. A married woman or a widow may be addressed as Mrs unless she has some other title or is known to prefer Ms. An unmarried woman may be addressed as Miss. There is a growing tendency to omit the title completely and simply use the name (Jill Smith or Omar Massoud) on the envelope. Other titles, such as Professor or Dr, should be used if appropriate.

— When writing a professional or business letter to a college, a company, an hotel, a professional journal, etc., the letter must be addressed to someone. You would, in fact, write to the Principal of a college, to the Secretary or Manager of a company, to the Manager or Receptionist of an hotel and to the Editor of a professional journal.

— The address follows the name, in this order:
  i. the number of the house and the name of the street (on the same line), *or* the name of the house (e.g. Allgoods Cottage) with the street name on a separate line
  ii. village, town or city
  iii. county (and country if written from abroad)
  iv. postal code.

For example:

    Ms C Gower
    116 Tenby Drive
    Fakenham
    Norfolk
    PE57 1ZZ

As can be seen from the above example, usual practice is to omit punctuation from the details of the name and address. On word-processed or typewritten letters, indentation is no longer used.

The letter

— The sender's address is written in full at the top right-hand side of the paper. It is not usual to put your name there. In care homes and hospitals and other places where official writing paper is printed, the address, including the telephone number and e-mail address, is either on the right-hand side or in the centre.

— In private letters the date is usually written below the sender's address in the order: day, month, year (e.g. 7 June 2006, or sometimes as 7.6.2006).

— In a professional or business letter, the name and address of the person to whom the letter is written are placed on the left-hand side, at the top, with the date written below the address.

— When you write to an unknown person the letter begins 'Dear Sir', or 'Dear Madam' if it is to a woman. If you are unsure, write 'Dear Sir/Madam'.

— When you have met the person or corresponded before, the last name is used and the letter begins with 'Dear Dr Sanchez'. If you know the person well or they have signed previous letters to you with their first name it is usual to address them by their first name (e.g. 'Dear Rao').

— When writing to a friend, one begins 'Dear John', 'Dear Farida', or 'My dear Elizabeth', to a closer friend.

— If the letter begins 'Dear Sir or Madam', the ending should be 'Yours faithfully'.

— If the letter begins, 'Dear Ms Steele' or some other name in a professional or business correspondence, the ending should be 'Yours sincerely'.

— 'With best wishes', 'With kindest regards' or 'Yours' are quite usual endings for letters to friends, or colleagues who you know well.

— Phrases such as 'Yours respectfully' are no longer used. Nor is it UK practice to use very flowery, effusive (over the top) language in a professional or business letter. Write clearly and simply and briefly in a professional or business letter.

— Each new subject or aspect of the subject should be dealt with in a separate paragraph. In a handwritten letter the paragraphs are marked by starting a little distance from the left side, or in word-processed letters by leaving space between the paragraphs.

— It is important to print your name in block letters underneath your signature, as names are often very difficult to read in handwriting. Also, note that in the UK the numbers one and seven are written thus: 1, 7. Figures written in the style used in continental European countries may cause delay, and even loss, to correspondence

— In situations where you have written asking for information such as details of a course, the institution may write to thank you for your interest and ask you to send an envelope with your address and enough postage stamps (stamped addressed envelope), so they can send you the printed material. The request for such an envelope is usually abbreviated to 'please send/enclose an SAE'.

Writing electronic mail

The use of electronic mail (e-mail) is increasingly important for both professional and private communication. The following list provides you with some guidance:

— Remember that e-mail cannot be 100% secure or confidential – it may be read by other people. It is especially important to make sure that e-mail containing patient/client details is only seen by those authorised to do so. Always follow the local protocols for keeping computer records confidential.

— It is important to be concise. People often get many e-mails each day and you want them to read yours.

— It is good sense to think before you send any written communication – you can change your mind right up to putting a letter in the postbox, but once you click on post/send for e-mail it is too late to change your mind. Feeling upset or angry is not an ideal time to send an e-mail.

— In common with professional or business letters, it is usual to address people as Mr, Ms, Mrs, Miss, Dr, etc., unless you know them well and generally use their first name.

— It is not appropriate to use e-mail abbreviations (e.g. 'BTW' for 'by the way') or nursing/medical abbreviations in professional e-mail. Not everyone will know what the abbreviation means, or an abbreviation may have more than one meaning.

— It is not necessary to overuse punctuation in e-mail, such as using many exclamation marks. It is much better to let your text emphasise the important points. Likewise, it is not usual to use upper case (capital) letters for whole words, as this is the e-mail equivalent to shouting.

— A reply is not always instant. It is important to remember that although e-mail usually reaches its destination in just a few minutes, it can take longer. Some people read and reply to their e-mail several times a day, but others may only check once a week.

REFERENCES

Nursing and Midwifery Council (NMC) 2002 Guidelines for records and record keeping. NMC, London.

FURTHER READING

Hoban V 2003 How to ... handle a handover. Nursing Times 99(9):54–55.

Communication in nursing

5

INTRODUCTION

Being able to communicate is an essential skill for all health professionals and it is particularly important for nurses who are with people and their families for many hours a day. It is not always easy to understand what people are saying or to get them to understand what you are trying to tell them. Sometimes nurses who qualified in the UK have difficulties understanding people who have regional accents and many patients use different words for feelings and everyday events. Some of these words are part of this chapter, and Chapter 6 (Colloquial English) gives you lots more examples.

Nurses need to communicate so they can find out about the people in their care by taking a nursing history, give them information about their care and teach them about managing their illness.

This chapter will help you with some of the questions needed to take a nursing history and plan care based on a commonly used Activities of Living Model of Nursing (see Roper et al 1996) and some other important nursing issues (e.g. confusion and anxiety). Short case histories that focus on a particular activity are included to help you with some common situations. There are extracts from dialogues (conversations) between nurses and people/clients/relatives that give you examples of what they may say to you in answer to your questions. These case histories will be useful when you deal with similar situations at work, and later reflect on the positive and negative features of a particular conversation you had with a patient/client and their family.

Note: All the people and case histories used are fictitious and are not based on any persons we have nursed or met when supervising students

GETTING STARTED

The first words you say to a person are very important – you need to get it right. You need to say who you are and why you are there. What you say will depend on the situation, but you might start with:

> 'Hello [or good morning/good evening] Mrs Jones I am Nurse [your last name/surname/family name].'

or just use your first and last names and say that you are the nurse who will be caring for them for the shift (or whatever is appropriate).

Ask Mrs Jones what she likes to be called. You will hear patients and nurses using lots of different forms of address; for example, the titles Mr, Ms, Miss, Mrs or Dr with the last name, or first names, or sometimes endearments such as love, dear, gran, nan, grandpa, honey, darling, mate, pet, hen, duck, etc. As a general rule it is not acceptable to use endearments when speaking to patients. Do not use a person's first name unless they ask you to do so. It is important to follow a person's wishes about their preferred form of address – make sure that this is written in the nursing notes for all nurses to read.

Once you know what the person wants to be called you can start to get the information needed to plan nursing care, explain the care, tests or treatment planned, and answer any questions. Remember that if you cannot answer a person's question it is important to get another nurse, doctor or other healthcare professional to do so.

Whenever possible ask simple questions that will ensure you get the exact information needed, and avoid using jargon. For example, saying to Mrs Jones 'I will be back to do your vital signs or obs' will mean nothing to her – you will need to explain that you will be back to record her blood pressure, temperature, pulse and respiration. Always check any prepared documents that arrive from the admissions office or the emergency department – the person's details may have changed or there might be a mistake.

Biographical data

— You will need to start with the assessment sheet, finding out details about your patient such as their full name, where they live (address) and who with.

> 'Mrs Jones can you tell me your full name [first name or forename followed by last name which is also called the surname or family name] and your address and telephone number.'

If you ask where they live patients might say 'In the town' or 'With my husband', so it is best to ask for the address (house number/name, the street, the town, county and the postcode, see Ch. 4). If you have problems spelling a name or address, always ask the patient or their relative to spell it out letter by letter or even copy it out for you – it must be accurate. It is important to ask your patient's age and date of birth, e.g. 57 years, 22/2/1946. In the UK dates are always written in the order day, month and year.

— Always ask the name and address of the patient's next of kin, and get telephone numbers (daytime and for use at night) in case it is necessary to contact family members. Obviously this might be necessary if the patient's condition worsens, but it might be to say that the person can come home so please can the family bring in outdoor clothes. If the next of kin lives many miles away the patient may give you contact details of a friend or neighbour (someone living close to them).

— An assessment includes asking about the patient's religion (if any) or spiritual needs, so you can plan care that ensures any religious, spiritual or cultural needs are met. These needs may include attending a religious service/ceremony, having a visit from a religious leader, priest, minister, mullah, rabbi, etc., or having facilities for prayer, needing to fast or having special food.

'What religion are you Mrs Jones?'

Then you can ask appropriate questions, such as

'Will you want to see your minister or visit the hospital chapel?'

In the UK many patients will answer with the abbreviation for their religion, e.g. 'C of E' for Church of England or 'RC' for Roman Catholic.

Work (employment) history

You will need to ask the patient if they work. This usually means paid work, but many people in the UK do unpaid voluntary work and this should also be recorded on the assessment form.

Once you know that the patient works you can get more details. The type of work may be influencing their health (e.g. exposure to substances such as asbestos that can cause cancer, work in a dusty environment and chest diseases, or back pain where heavy objects must be moved). The length of time off work following an operation will depend on the type of work the patient does, and in some situations patients cannot go back to their old job (e.g. some driving jobs following a heart attack (myocardial infarction)).

The question:

'What do you do?'

usually means 'What is your work?'. Patients may tell you where they work (i.e. the company name) rather than the type of job they do. So if they say

'I've been at Clarks since I left school and that's nearly 30 years'

you will have to ask:

'What job do you do at Clarks?'

'Do you work full time or part time?'

'How many hours do you work in a week?'

'Do you work shifts?' (This relates to irregular hours, e.g. in a hospital or factory.)

'How long have you been doing this job?'

'Do you have a stressful job? 'Do you work late or have to take work home?'

If patients are not working you need to find out why – are they retired from work and, if so, ask what type of work they used to do, looking after children or a relative, looking for work, studying or unable to work for health reasons.

Reason for admission or contact with health services and medical details

— *The patient's understanding of reason for admission/treatment, etc*. It is important to find out exactly why the patient thinks they have visited the general practitioner/practice nurse, or come into hospital or the care home. It might be correct to ask a direct question such as:

'What do you think is the matter with you?'

or

'Tell me why you have come in today.'

This last type of comment might be used for a patient coming in for a planned operation. The patient may say something like

'I've come in to get my cataract done [operated on].'

Sometimes you will need to use questions such as:

'Have you been having some problems at home?'

and the patient may say:

'I've been having dizzy turns [vertigo] when I keel over [fall over].'

or

'I had a spell [a period of time] of feeling very down [depressed mood] but that has cleared up [got better, disappeared] now.'

You will also need to check that the family know why the patient has been admitted.

— *Past medical history and family history.* You will need to ask about past illnesses or operations. For example, a patient coming in for a routine operation may have type 1 diabetes or they may have severe arthritis that makes walking very difficult and you will need to plan care accordingly. You might ask:

'Have you ever had any serious illnesses in the past?'

'Have you ever had an operation?'

'Have you ever been in hospital before?'

'Have you ever had any accidents or injuries?'

'Is there anything else you'd like to tell me?

As some illnesses, such as some types of heart disease and diabetes, may run in certain families (familial) you will also need to ask about the family medical history:

'Are there any serious illnesses in you family?'

— *Allergies.* Always ask about any allergies, including foods, drugs (see below) and other substances such as washing powders:

'Are you allergic to anything?'

'Have you any allergies?'

It might be necessary to ask the family, for example, if the patient is a child, has dementia or is unconscious.

— *Drugs.* It is necessary to ask all patients/clients if they are taking any drugs, but it is worth remembering that some patients will associate the word 'drugs' with illegal substances and drug misuse, so you can ask:

'Are you taking any medicines (or drugs)?'

Always ask patients about all types of drugs, including those prescribed by a doctor or nurse, drugs they buy at the chemist (pharmacy) or supermarket (over-the-counter drugs), natural remedies such as St. John's Wort, and if appropriate ask about recreational (illegal) drugs such as cannabis. It is vital to know about any drug allergies (e.g. penicillin) or adverse drug reactions. Always ask and make sure that this is recorded in all the relevant nursing documentation.

Physical function and effects of current illness on daily living or work

Many areas of physical function, such as mobility (moving about), are covered in the dialogue section (see pp. 59–123), but you will need to ask how the current illness affects everyday life.

For example:

'Is there anything you need help with at home, such as getting out of bed or making a cup of tea?'

'How often does your neighbour come in to help you?'

'Are you still able to work?'

Social history

— *Support networks* are important particularly after discharge. You can ask questions that include:

'Do your family live close by?'

'Who will be at home to look after you when you are discharged?'

'Will you be able to stay with your family until you are able to manage back at home?'

— *Type of home.* Although you know the patient's address, you also need to know about the type of home they have. Patients who live alone in a big house may be unable to keep it heated or clean after discharge, and a patient who lives in a flat up several flights of stairs may need to be found a ground-floor flat before they can go home. You will need to ask questions that include:

'Do you live in a house, bungalow, flat, bedsit, etc.?'

(A bedsit is a room used for both sleeping and daytime activities with the use of shared kitchen and bathroom.)

'How do you heat your home?'

(Patients may not be able to manage an open fire or may not use expensive heating if they are living on a low wage, pension or benefits.)

'Do you have good neighbours?'

(The patient may be relying on the neighbours to check the house, feed pets, take in post and do things like cutting the grass while they are in hospital.)

— *Social problems due to present condition/admission.* Patients admitted as an emergency may be worried about children or others such as older relatives at home who depend on them. Many people in the UK have pet animals such as a cat or dog and you should always ask if they have a pet, and if someone is caring for them.

'Do you have any pets at home?'

'What's your cat's name?'

'Who is feeding Harry?'

You will need to listen very carefully, as a patient with dementia, for example, may keep repeating the name of the pet animal rather than tell you the details. Patients can be very anxious about the care of their pet animals while they are in hospital or a care home.

— *Hobbies and interests.*

'How do you spend your free time?'

'How much exercise do you take?'

'Do you play any sports?'

'Have you any hobbies?'

'Do you like to watch TV [television] or listen to music?'

— *Contacts with and input from other health and social care professionals.* Many older patients will already be in contact with a wide range of health and social care professions, such as a district nurse, health visitor, practice nurse, general practitioner (family doctor), physiotherapist, occupational therapist, speech and language therapist, dietician, podiatrist or social worker. You should ask about this and find out who comes, how often and what they do:

'Do you see the nurse at home?'

'What do the nurses do?'

'Do they come in everyday?'

Lifestyle

During the nursing assessment you will need to find out about lifestyle or behaviour that can influence health in both good or bad ways (e.g. the type of foods eaten, amount of exercise, alcohol intake, use of drugs, use of tobacco, sexual behaviour and high-risk leisure activities). Often a person's lifestyle or behaviour is sensitive and they may feel embarrassed or guilty if you ask lots of questions. Thus direct questioning does not always work well in this situation, but often you will be able to get the information as the patient talks about their lifestyle and view of health. For example, a patient may tell you, without any prompting, that they know they do not get enough exercise and you can find out more by asking them what they mean. Sometimes, however, you will need to ask more directly and the sort of questions that may be needed to get information about some of these lifestyle issues are discussed in the following section under the related activity.

BREATHING

Some nursing/medical or Standard English words and corresponding colloquial words and expressions associated with breathing are given in Box 5.1.

Note: Colloquial expressions used in the case histories and example conversations are explained in brackets [...].

Box 5.1 Words associated with breathing (for further examples see Ch. 6)	
Nursing/medical or Standard English words	Colloquial (everyday) or slang (very informal) words and expressions used by patients
Dyspnoea	Breathlessness; out of breath; puffed; short of breath; fighting for breath (severe cases)
Expectorate	To bring up/cough up phlegm; spit
Expiration	Breathing out
Inhaler for drugs	Puffer
Inspiration	Breathing in
Respiration	Breathing
Sputum	Phlegm (pronounced *flem*)

Case history – Mr and Mrs Ryan

Mr Ryan has been admitted to the medical assessment unit with a chest infection causing an exacerbation [worsening] of his chronic obstructive pulmonary disease (COPD). He is very distressed and finding it hard to breathe. His wife tells you that 'His breathing has been bad for years and he can't get about much these days' – meaning that his mobility is reduced. You can get the biographical data from Mrs Ryan, and as soon as Mr Ryan's condition improves you can find out more about his breathing and related problems. You might also want to ask Mrs Ryan if her husband becomes confused or mixed up [disorientated], as this may be a sign of reduced oxygen getting to the brain (caused by hypoxia), or if he is more drowsy [sleepy] than normal. This may happen if there is too much carbon dioxide in the arterial blood (hypercapnia).

Nurse: Mrs Ryan have you noticed a change in your husband's mental state recently, does he get confused?

Mrs R.:	Now you come to mention it he does seem a bit dotty [silly] sometimes. You know, not always knowing where he is.
Nurse:	**Hello Mr Ryan tell me about the problems you have with your breathing.**
Mr R.:	I'm breathless most of the time but the infection made it much worse – I was really frightened and felt that I was fighting for breath until the treatment (more bronchodilators, corticosteroids and antibiotic therapy) started to work [became effective].
Nurse:	**Before the infection how was your breathing? Were you breathless sitting still?**
Mr R.:	Oh no, only when I tried to walk about.
Nurse:	**Can you normally get upstairs in one go [without stopping]?**
Mr R.:	Only if I rest on the landing [flat part of a staircase] and get my breath back [recover].
Nurse:	**How far can you walk on the level without getting breathless?**
Mr R.:	I can get as far as the back garden but I'm fair jiggered [exhausted, breathless] after.
Nurse:	**Is there anything else about your breathing? Do you wheeze [make an audible noise when breathing]?**
Mr R.:	Yes, I do wheeze and my chest often feels tight, but Dr Singh is going to put me on something new [prescribe a different drug], so hopefully that will do the trick [hopes the new treatment will be effective] – fingers crossed [hope for good luck].
Nurse:	**Hope so. What medicines were you taking at home before you came into the ward?**
Mr R.:	The blue inhaler [salbutamol inhaler], and the antibiotics from the GP for the infection.
Nurse:	**Are you using oxygen at home?**
Mr R.:	Yes, for up to 15 hours a day. It's OK, we have a machine that takes some gases out of the air and leaves the oxygen [oxygen concentrator] for me, so the

	missus [wife] doesn't need to keep changing cylinders and I can get around in the house and out as far as the back garden.
Nurse:	**What else helps your breathing?**
Mr R.:	Well – sitting up and leaning on the table helps, but when I'm very chesty [trouble with chest, coughing] it's better to sleep downstairs in an armchair. At least the wife gets some sleep even if I don't. A while ago I started doing relaxation exercises and that helps when I feel panicky [frightened], but they didn't work last night – worse luck.
Nurse:	**Do you still smoke?**
Mr R.:	No, not for years.
Nurse:	**When did you stop smoking?**
Mr R.:	I used to smoke roll-ups [cigarettes that the patient makes himself] and I cut myself down [reduced the number of cigarettes] to 10 a day, and then I said 'That's it. No more' and I haven't smoked for 5 years. It was hard but I was determined to stick to [keep to] no smoking.
Nurse:	**That's good, but do you still cough?**
Mr R.:	Yes, cough and bring up stuff [phlegm or sputum]. I had a smokers' cough [early morning cough] when I was in the Army, but now I cough any time of the day or night.
Nurse:	**What colour is the sputum you cough up? Has the amount increased?**
Mr R.:	Really green because of the infection, and much more, and my mouth tastes foul.
Nurse:	**We sent a specimen to the laboratory earlier, so I'll get you some sputum pots and tissues and some mouthwash. The physiotherapist is on his way up to see you, so he will help you to cough and clear your chest. Do you have any pain with the cough?**
Mr R.:	Not at the moment.
Nurse:	**What about washing and dressing – are you able to manage**

	or do you need some help?
Mr R.:	Just need some help to wash my back and feet. She does it at home [meaning Mrs Ryan helps].
Nurse:	**How is your appetite? What about eating and drinking?**
Mr R.:	I'm trying to have a drink every hour like you said, but I can't face [manage] a big meal.
Nurse:	**I will ask the dietician to visit and discuss it with you, but for today I can give you some nourishing drinks and order snacks or light meals for you.**
Mr R.:	Thanks, that sounds spot on [exactly right].
Nurse:	**Your bed is close to the bathroom and lavatory. Will you be able to walk or will a wheelchair be easier?**
Mr R.:	It's not far – I can get there, but after washing I might need some help back.
Nurse:	**How are you sleeping?**
Mr R.:	Don't worry I'll sleep OK tonight – after today with having to call the ambulance and everything I'm knackered [exhausted].
Nurse:	**Is there anything you would like to ask me?**
Mr R.:	No thanks. You and the doctor explained what was going on [happening] earlier and I do understand about COPD. An 'expert patient' you might say.
Nurse:	**Just ring the bell if you need me. I think Mrs Ryan went to phone your son and have a cup of tea while we did the paperwork. I'll bring her in to you when she gets back.**

Other questions

Mr Ryan will find it difficult to talk for long if he is breathless, so you may need to ask some other questions later. Sometimes it will not be necessary to ask because Mr Ryan may tell you extra things as you are attending to his care or he may tell other health professionals, such as the physiotherapist.

Other questions may include some of the following:

'Do you have pain or chest discomfort on breathing or coughing?'

'Do your ankles get swollen?'

'Is there anything that makes you cough worse, such as a smoky or dusty atmosphere, or changes in temperature like going out into the cold? Does any position make it worse?'

'Have you noticed any blood in your sputum?' Is there a lot of blood or is it streaked with blood?

COMMUNICATING

Some nursing/medical or Standard English words and corresponding colloquial words and expressions associated with communicating are given in Box 5.2.

Note: Colloquial expressions used in the case histories and example conversations are explained in brackets [...].

Box 5.2 Words associated with communicating (for further examples see Ch. 6)	
Nursing/medical or Standard English words	Colloquial (everyday) or slang (very informal) words and expressions used by patients
Diplopia	Double vision; seeing double
Dysarthria	Can't get the words out
Dysphasia (aphasia)	I know what to say but nothing comes out; I can't find the right word; the sentence comes out all wrong; I can say the word but I don't know what it means
Hearing impairment, deafness	Hard of hearing; deaf as a post
Tinnitus	Ringing, buzzing or roaring sound in the ears
Visual impairment, blindness	Can't see the hand in front of me; blind as a bat
Vertigo	Dizzy; dizziness; giddy

Case history – Mrs Egbewole

Mrs Egbewole had a stroke (cerebrovascular accident) about 18 months ago, and her family, with the help of twice-daily visits from the home carer, usually look after her at home. She has come into the care home while her family has a short holiday. The stroke has left Mrs Egbewole with left-sided paralysis and poor balance. She does not have dysphasia, but because the left side of her face is also paralysed she sometimes has slurred speech and dribbles saliva. She also has problems with non-verbal communication because her facial expression is affected.

Nurse: Mrs Egbewole, do you have any problems with your speech?

Mrs E.: It is slurred sometimes, but that's because my mouth doesn't work properly.

Nurse: How does that make you feel?

Mrs E.: I feel really embarrassed, especially if I'm talking to someone new.

Nurse: How can we help?

Mrs E.: I'll be all right as long as [provided] people give me enough time to get the words out. It gets me flustered [agitated/confused] if people are impatient'

Nurse: I'll make sure that is recorded in your care plan and that all members of staff know to give you plenty of time to tell us things. Did you see the speech and language therapist after the stroke?'

Mrs E.: Yes, but I couldn't handle it [cope] so soon after losing my husband [my husband died].

Nurse: How would you feel about trying again with speech and language therapy?

Mrs E.: If you think it might help I'm willing to give it another go [try again].

Nurse: Fine – I'll organise a referral. Is there anything else that's troubling you?

Mrs E.: Well yes there is, and it's all down to [caused by] the muscles in my face not working properly. I can't help dribbling [saliva flows from the mouth].

Nurse: You obviously know about keeping the skin round your mouth clean and dry because there is no sign of soreness.

Mrs E.: Yes, the nurses on the stroke unit really stressed good skin care. But another thing that worries me is the look of my face – it's really lopsided [asymmetrical] and when I try to smile I must look dreadful.

Nurse: Maybe the speech and language therapist can suggest something to help, but you could mention it to Dr Newell. She will be in this afternoon.

Mrs E.: That's a good idea – I will add it to my list of questions I have for her.

Nurse: How is your sight? I see you have spectacles/glasses on at the moment.

Mrs E.: Yes, I'm blind as a bat without them [usually meaning poor vision rather than completely blind] and have needed help for years. I used to have contact lenses, but after my stroke I found it too difficult to take them out, so I got some specs [short for 'spectacles'].

Nurse: Do you have a second pair for reading or does the one pair do for everything?

Mrs E.: They are bifocals and I am supposed to look through a different bit for reading. But if the print is very small, such as on food labels, I use a magnifying glass instead.

Nurse: Did you bring the magnifying glass in with you?

Mrs E.: Oh yes, my carer packed everything but the kitchen sink [implies that the carer was very thorough when he packed Mrs Egbewole's suitcase].

Nurse: Who normally cleans your spectacles?

Mrs E.: My lovely [meaning admirable in this case] carers do that, I can't with only one good hand.

Nurse: Would you like me to give them a clean now?

Mrs E.: Thanks – they're not very clean and it makes things look blurred.

Nurse: Do you have any other problems with your eyes? Sometimes a stroke can affect vision, such as seeing things double.

Mrs E.:   Oh no, I was lucky [that the stroke did not affect her sight]. When I was younger I suffered terribly [very badly affected] with migraine and then I used to see flashing lights with a zigzag pattern before the headache came on [started]. If I'm out in a cold wind my eyes start running [watering; tears flow down the cheeks], but that's normal.

Nurse: **Definitely normal – it certainly happens to me.**

Case history – Mr Sandford

Mr Sandford is 42 years old and has poor hearing, tinnitus and problems with the build-up of earwax, which also affects his hearing. He has Down syndrome and lives independently at the local group housing complex where he has a bedsit. He works full-time in a supermarket. His parents are dead, but his two older sisters, who live close by, see him several times a week and he has many friends from work and in the house.

Nurse: **Hello Mr Sandford, I'm Nurse MacGregor. I understand that you have come to see us about your hearing.**

Mr S.:   Hello, everyone calls me Nick. My hearing is no good, I can't hear them on the telly [television] or the boss [manager] at the shop.

Nurse: **Can you hear me all right?**

Mr S.:   Yes.

Nurse: **What would you like me to call you?**

Mr S.:   You can call me Nick if you like.

Nurse: **OK. Has your hearing always been bad Nick?'**

Mr S.:   Not as bad – it's really bad now and I can't hear the telly.

Nurse: **What do you like on the telly?**

Mr S.:   I watch Eastenders and Coronation Street [both popular, long-running series in the UK], they're the best and I like the football as well.

Nurse: **What helps you to hear?**

Mr S.:   Like now when I can see you and nobody else is talking. When I'm calm.

Nurse: Anything else?

Mr S.: The ear wash [ear irrigation, previously known as 'syringing'] but it feels funny [strange].

Nurse: We can have a look inside your ears with the special light [otoscope] to check for wax, you might need another ear wash to help you hear.

Mr S.: OK.

Nurse: Have you got a hearing aid?

Mr S.: Don't like it.

Nurse: What don't you like?

Mr S.: It's broken.

Nurse: Have you got it with you? Perhaps the technician can mend it.

Mr S.: Here it is, but it's no good.

Nurse: I'll take it to the technician in a bit [in a short while]. Does anything else happen as well as not being able to hear?

Mr S.: Roaring [loud noise] and buzzing [like the sound made by insects] in my ears.

Nurse: Anything else?

Mr S.: My ears feel stuffed up [fullness] and I get giddy [experience vertigo] and stagger.

Nurse: Do you fall over?

Mr S.: I know it's coming, so I sit down.

SAFETY AND PREVENTING ACCIDENTS

Some nursing/medical or Standard English words and corresponding colloquial words and expressions associated with safety and preventing accidents are given in Box 5.3.

Note: Colloquial expressions used in the case histories and example conversations are explained in brackets […].

Case history – Mrs Kaur

Mrs Kaur has scalded her arm while making a cup of tea. Her neighbour brought her to the Emergency Department after they

Box 5.3   Words associated with safety and preventing accidents
(for further examples see Ch. 6)

Nursing/medical or Standard English words	Colloquial (everyday) or slang (very informal) words and expressions used by patients
Fall	Took a tumble; lost my footing; tripped up
Fracture	Broken or cracked (as in bone)
Seizure	Fit; funny turn; convulsion; an attack
Sprain	Twisted (as in ankle)
Syncope	Fainting attack; black out; collapse; pass out
Unconscious	Knocked out (KO'd); out cold; dead to the world; out of it

had bathed the damaged area with lots of cool water and kept it cool on the way to hospital with a wet towel. She is upset about being so clumsy and feels that she has been a nuisance to her neighbour and to the hospital staff who already have enough to do. Luckily the skin damage is superficial and should be completely healed in a few days.

Nurse: Hello again Mrs Kaur. Have the painkillers worked [taken away the pain]?

Mrs K.:   Hello Nurse. Yes, the pain is much less. My arm just feels sore [tender].

Nurse: The plan is to keep the scald dry and warm and let it heal. I've come to put a dressing on your arm.

Mrs K.:   I don't want anything that will stick.

Nurse: The dressings we use don't stick anymore, they are made to be non-adherent.

Mrs K.:   I remember the pain years ago when dressings did stick.

Nurse: The dressing only needs to be on for a few days and the scald will heal. It was a good thing that you knew the first aid for scalds, cooling the skin down certainly stopped it getting any worse.

Mrs K.: I saw a thing on the telly [television] about what to do with burns. But what about some burn ointment? It must need something.

Nurse: If you leave the dressing on for 2 or 3 days the scald will heal without any other treatment. You can take mild painkillers such as paracetamol if your arm is sore.

Mrs K.: I don't like the idea of taking it [the dressing] off myself.

Nurse: Well today is Saturday, so it should all be healed by Monday. You can get an appointment with the practice nurse for Tuesday and she can take off the dressing and check your arm.

Mrs K.: Sounds sensible – I will do that. I really feel such a fool – how could I pour boiling water over myself. I am doing all the silly things my granny [grandmother] did when she was 80.

Nurse: How do you think it happened?

Mrs K.: I can't seem to judge where the cup is. It's the same when I pour orange juice into a glass. And the kettle is so heavy.

Nurse: Have you had your eyes checked recently?

Mrs K.: My routine test must be due very soon – I will phone on Monday.

Nurse: Could you talk to the practice nurse about the trouble [difficulty] you have when pouring fluids?

Mrs K.: Yes, do you think I should tell her about how things are blurred and sometimes lines look very odd and wavy?

Nurse: That sounds like a good idea. But what can you do to make the kettle easier to use?

Mrs K.: I forget it's only me having a drink and usually fill it too full.

Nurse: Yes, I just fill mine without thinking. I have seen smaller kettles. Perhaps you would find that easier.

Mrs K.: My daughter can get me one when she goes to the big shops.

Case history – Mr Anderson

Mr Anderson is going home with several different drugs. He has been in hospital to have intravenous antibiotics for cellulitis and needs to have a course of oral antibiotics (phenoxymethylpenicillin, flucloxacillin and metronidazole). He also takes an antiepileptic drug (sodium valproate) to control generalised seizures and a diuretic (torasemide) for hypertension.

Nurse: The antibiotics for you to take home have come up from the pharmacy and I would like to go over [discuss] what you need to do. There are instructions on the labels, but it helps if we talk it through [discuss] as well.

Mr A.: Yeah [yes], OK then. I want to get it right. It was a bit of a fright ending up in here just for a cat bite gone septic [infected].

Nurse: What seems like such a minor thing can quickly get really bad. There are three separate antibiotics to take – here look [at the containers]. There are two penicillins: flucloxacillin and phenoxymethylpenicillin. You need to take these every 6 hours and an hour before food or on an empty stomach. These are the best ones for your infection and you have already told us that you are not allergic to penicillin. The other antibiotic is metronidazole, which you need to take every 8 hours, but this time with or after food.

Mr A.: Yeah, no problems with penicillin and I'm used to taking tablets – with the Epilim [a proprietary name for sodium valproate] twice a day and the Torem [proprietary name for torasemide] first thing [early morning].

Nurse: Will there be any problem with having to take two before food and one with or after food?

Mr A.: No, I already need to remember to take the Epilim after food.

Nurse: What about writing out a chart? That would help, especially if you cross off doses as you take them.

Mr A.: I don't write so well, but one of our kids [children] can do it.

Nurse: It is important to take the antibiotics at regular times and to finish the 7-day course even if your hand seems better.

Mr A.: Why can't I stop once it looks better?

Nurse: Finishing the course means that the treatment will kill off all the bugs [bacteria in this case] – the infection is cured, and it is very important the bugs don't become immune [develop resistance] to the antibiotics.

Mr A.: What like that MRSA has? OK. I'll carry on [continue] to the end.

Nurse: Yes, just like MRSA, but you haven't got that. There are a few other things I need to tell you about the metronidazole. It is important to swallow the tablets whole with plenty of water. And you shouldn't drink alcohol while you are taking them and for 2 days after you stop – it can cause a nasty reaction with nausea and sickness [vomiting]. You might have a furred tongue and your urine can be dark.

Mr A.: That's a blow [disappointment]. I could really do with a couple of pints [meaning he would enjoy some beer]. Thanks for the warning about my pee [urine]. That would have really put the wind up me [alarm me].

Nurse: Have you got plenty of Epilim and Torem at home?

Mr A.: Yeah – I never run out of tablets [have none left]. I dread having another fit [seizure] now that they have settled down.

Nurse: Have you any questions or bits you don't quite understand?

Mr A.: It's a lot to take in [information to absorb, understand]. Can you go through it all again please?

Nurse: You're right it is a lot of information. Let's start with the three antibiotics and when to take them ...

MOBILITY

Some nursing/medical or Standard English words and correspon-ding colloquial words and expressions associated with mobility

Box 5.4 Words associated with mobility (for further examples see Ch. 6)	
Nursing/medical or Standard English words	Colloquial (everyday) or slang (very informal) words and expressions used by patients
Akinesia	Freezing or frozen; rooted to the spot; can't go forward
Ataxia	Staggering; jerky; shaky; all over the place
Bradykinesia	Can't get started; slowed me almost to a halt; slowed me down nearly to a complete stop
Dorsal part of a phalangeal joint, especially the meta-carpophalangeal joints (with fingers flexed)	Knuckle
Sudden tonic muscle contraction	Cramp
Festination	Shuffling; can't stop once I get going
Swollen	Puffed up
Swollen and deformed (as an arthritic finger joint)	Knobbly
Tremor	The shakes

are given in Box 5.4.

Note: Colloquial expressions used in the case histories and example conversations are explained in brackets [...].

Case history – Ms Wayne

Joint stiffness and pain are causing Ms Wayne severe difficulties with mobility. She has had rheumatoid arthritis for many years and now has some joint destruction and deformity with associated muscle wasting. At the moment she feels generally unwell – very lethargic, her temperature is slightly elevated and she has anorexia. In the past she has had surgery to her hands, which are very badly affected.

Ms W.: Hello Nurse. Have you sorted out [organised] my physiotherapy appointment yet?

Nurse: **Yes, the physiotherapist is coming to treat you here. What do they usually do?**

Ms W.: In the past I had heat treatment, but now they concentrate on gentle exercise and making sure that my hand splints are still helping and not making my skin sore.

Nurse: **Tell me how your mobility is affected by the arthritis.**

Ms W.: I have trouble [difficulties] getting in and out of bed, or the bath, and I need help to get out of a low chair.

Nurse: **What about walking?**

Ms W.: Getting about [moving about, going out] is hard. I get around the house with the walking aid and tend to use a wheelchair when I go out. The car has been modified so at least I'm independent. I can go shopping and out with my pals [friends].

Nurse: **Yes, that is important.**

Ms W.: I'm not going to be an invalid [someone who is always ill], always needing help and griping [complaining] about the unfairness of it all.

Nurse: **How do you stay so positive?**

Ms W.: After my joints, especially my hands, got really bad [deteriorated] and I had to give up work [left employment] I thought 'I'm only 40 and can't just do nothing'. So I looked at ways I could be busy and useful.

Nurse: **What do you do?**

Ms W.: I go into the local primary school three mornings a week and listen to the children read. It's a great [good] feeling when you hear them improve and become more confident. Just lately I started helping on a telephone helpline for people with disabilities – there are special hands-free phones so I don't need to use my hands much.

Nurse: We [meaning Ms Wayne and the nurse] can sort out your care plan now and make sure that we include the help you need. You must tell me your usual routine for the hand splints, as you're the expert. Can you arrange for your own wheelchair to be brought in?

Ms W.:   My brother can fetch it at lunchtime if I give him a ring [contact by telephone].

Nurse: What about other activities? Do you have difficulty using your hands?

Ms W.:   Yes, the pain and stiffness in my hands and wrists really hold me back [curb or inhibit]. My hands look so awful with the finger joints all puffed up [swollen] and it's so frustrating and it really riles [annoys, makes me angry] me when I can't do something simple like doing up [fastening] buttons. It's always worse in the morning when you need to wash and dress, which is a real pain [nuisance] when I'm due at the school.

Nurse: Are there any other movements that you find difficult?

Ms W.:   Anything where I have to grip and move my wrist like holding the kettle and pouring.

Nurse: Again we can plan what help you will need from us while you're here. Do you see the OT [occupational therapist] for help with this?

Ms W.:   Yes, she has been so helpful – lots of gadgets to help me do things, like dressing and cooking, for myself, and so many good ideas about how to do things without getting tired or making the pain worse.

Nurse: Perhaps your brother can bring in the gadgets you need in here when he comes with the wheelchair. What do you think?

Ms W.:   OK. I hadn't thought of that.

Nurse: The rheumatology nurse specialist will be up later to

> review your drugs with Dr Wong [the rheumatologist], and co-ordinate all the other practitioners – I expect you know them both quite well by now.

Ms W.: Yes, I certainly do. Having Sam [Ms Wayne has known the nurse specialist for several years and they use first names] is a real support – he's always there on the phone and it's so nice to see the same person at the nurse-led clinics. I'm a bit disappointed about the new drugs we tried – the benefits have definitely worn off [become less effective].

Nurse: **Do you need anything for pain?**

Ms W.: No, not at the moment thanks. I took all my morning drugs at home and I'd rather wait to see what happens after the drug review.

Case history – Mr Lajowski

Mr Lajowski has come into the day-surgery unit to have a lipoma removed from his back. His mobility is seriously affected by Parkinson's disease, which he has had for some years. He is not particularly anxious about the surgery, as this was explained to him at the pre-admission assessment clinic, but he is worried about how he will cope with moving about in the new environment.

Nurse: **Hello Mr Lajowski. I understand that you have come in today to have a fatty lump [lipoma] removed from your back and the plan is to send you home later this afternoon.**

Mr L.: Yes, that's right. The lump needs to come off [be removed] – it gets in the way of the waistband of my trousers. I shall be glad to see the back of it [pleased when it has gone]. Did they tell you that I have Parkinson's disease?

Nurse: **Yes, it's in your notes from the assessment clinic. How does it affect you?**

Mr L.: The walking is the worst. Its difficult to start moving and I'm so slow [bradykinesia]. All I can do is shuffle [feet sliding, legs dragging, characteristic of Parkinson's disease] to start with and then my steps get shorter and I get faster and faster [festination], can't stop, and like as not [likely] over I go [fall over]. I've really lost my nerve [to lose confidence]. If you saw me you would think I was the worse for drink ['drink' in this case means alcoholic drink – the person is drunk, or intoxicated, or inebriated].

Nurse:	**Do you have any other movement problems?**
Mr L.:	I get that freezing [akinesia] where I'm rooted to the spot [can't move]. It mostly comes on out of the blue [comes unexpectedly], but I worked it out [found out, realised] that trying to do more than one thing at once [simultaneously] will bring it on [cause it]. The shaking [tremor] in my hands is bad, and its hard to do some things because my arms are so stiff [caused by rigidity].
Nurse:	**What things are particularly difficult for you?**
Mr L.:	It sounds daft [absurd], but it's mainly things like turning over in bed, reaching out for a cup, getting up out of a chair and turning round once I'm up.
Nurse:	**Are there things that help?**
Mr L.:	I've learnt a few tricks [ways to overcome the problems], such as having a good firm mattress and a high-backed chair with arms. The others things are really simple, like other people waiting until I'm ready to move and giving me time to do things for myself. When I freeze, the physio' [physiotherapist] told me to try stepping over an imaginary line, or to count 'one–two' out loud with each step and that does help.
Nurse:	**What about other activities, such as those needing fine movements?**
Mr L.:	Doing up [fastening] shoelaces or buttons is impossible, so that material that sticks to itself is very handy [helpful, useful]. What's it called again?
Nurse:	**Oh, you mean Velcro. It's very useful, we use it a lot in the rehab. [rehabilitation] unit.**

Mr L.:   I get loads [a lot] of cramp [sudden tonic muscle contraction] attacks at night, so I'm awake half the night [disturbed sleep]. Before the Parkinson's I could just pop out [get out] of bed and it would go.

Nurse: Not so easy now.

Mr L.:   How right you are. I wish it would settle down [become quiescent].

Nurse: I gather [understand] that your medication has just [recently] been changed.

Mr L.:   Yes, I said to the Doc [short for doctor] that the cramp had gone on [continued] too long and he said that I could try some different tablets.

Nurse: Any luck with the new tablets [meaning are they effective]?

Mr L.:   Early days [too soon to be sure], but I think the cramps have eased off [become less frequent].

EATING AND DRINKING

Some nursing/medical or Standard English words and corresponding colloquial words and expressions associated with eating and drinking are given in Box 5.5.

Note: Colloquial expressions used in the case histories and example conversations are explained in brackets […].

Case history – Miss Hyde-Whyte

Miss Hyde-Whyte has come into the community hospital for assessment. She lives alone and has been retired for over 20 years. The district nursing team, who have been visiting Miss Hyde-Whyte to treat her leg ulcer, have recently become concerned about her lack of interest in meals and obvious weight loss.

Nurse: Hello Miss Hyde-Whyte, I'm Nurse Mosquera. I would like to ask you some questions. Will that be all right?

Miss H.:   Hello – please call me Maggie. The rest is such a mouthful [difficult to say].

Box 5.5 Words associated with eating and drinking (for further examples see Ch. 6)

Nursing/medical or Standard English words	Colloquial (everyday) or slang (very informal) words and expressions used by patients
Abdomen	Belly; gut; stomach; tummy
Abdominal pain	Belly ache; gut rot; stomach/tummy ache
Anorexia	No appetite
Dyspepsia	Acid indigestion; heartburn
Good appetite	Always hungry; eat like a horse; ready for my grub
Halitosis	Bad breath; mouth odour
Nausea	Biliousness; feel sick; queasiness
Oesophagus	Gullet
Poor appetite	Can't face food; don't eat enough to keep a bird alive; been off my food; not hungry; peck or pick at food
Stomatitis	Mouth ulcers; sore mouth
Vomit	Be sick; bring up; lose the lot; puke; retch; sick up; spew; throw up

---

Nurse: I will need to weigh you and measure your height, but first a few questions.

Miss H.: I'm sure that I have lost weight – all my clothes hang on me [are much too big].

Nurse: How often do you eat and drink?

Miss H.: Well I used to have breakfast, a proper cooked lunch and something on toast or a sandwich in the evening.

Nurse: Has something changed?

Miss H.: I used to really enjoy cooking, have a G&T [gin and tonic] and then sit at the table with a nice meal, but now I've got no appetite and I just pick at it [the food]. My dad [father] would have said you don't eat enough to keep a bird alive [have a poor appetite].

Nurse: **Why do you think your appetite has decreased?**

Miss H.: Two reasons I think. I've had mouth ulcers for ages [a long time]. Probably my false teeth [dentures] don't fit anymore; and I have been sick [vomited] a few times after meals.

Nurse: **I'll look at your mouth in a moment [in a short time] and see if any treatment would help. It might be a good idea to see your dentist about the poorly fitting dentures. Tell me about the vomiting.**

Miss H.: If I eat a proper meal I soon feel sick [nauseated] and then I'm sick [vomit]. The food just comes back.

Nurse: **Are you sick at any other time?**

Miss H.: No, only after food.

Nurse: **What colour is the vomit? Is there any blood or bile?**

Miss H.: No blood and it's not green or yellow like bile. The colour varies – it depends on what I've eaten.

Nurse: **Sometimes blood can look like coffee grounds [describes the appearance of partially digested blood in the vomit] – anything like that?**

Miss H.: No, nothing like that.

Nurse: **How do you feel afterwards?**

Miss H.: That's the strange thing. Once I've been sick I feel fine [all right]. My stomach [abdomen] feels uncomfortable before I'm sick, but that feeling soon goes afterwards.

Nurse: **When you were eating normally what sort of food did you cook?**

Miss H.: Proper meals – meat or fish and lots of veg. [short for 'vegetables'] and I always had dessert or some cheese. No point doing all that if you're going to be sick.

Nurse: **How often do you usually shop for food?**

Miss H.: Most days. It's nice to get out and have a chat [talk] with people.

Nurse: **What do you eat and drink now?**

Miss H.: I know that I must eat something, so I have things like scrambled [a cooking method] egg on toast, soup and milky drinks. It's not unpleasant [In English when you have two negatives, known as a 'double negative', it creates a middle way, meaning 'not a positive' ('a pleasant diet') but not a negative ('an unpleasant diet') either. So here, 'not unpleasant' means a fairly acceptable diet], but I know it's not enough.

Nurse: **Let's see how much you weigh. What's your normal weight?**

Miss H.: Before the vomiting started I had been about 10 stone [an Imperial Unit of weight where 1 stone = 14 pounds, see Ch. 11] for as long as I can remember [for a long time].

Nurse: **We use the kilogram for weight, but I can tell what it is in stones and pounds.**

Miss H.: What's the verdict [finding] then. Have I lost much?

Nurse: **I'm afraid [The phrase 'I'm afraid', is used to introduce news which is unwelcome or bad] you have lost about 11 kilograms. You weigh 52 kilograms; that's 8 stone 2 pounds, so that's nearly 2 stone less than usual. We will have to keep an eye on [keep a frequent check] your weight.**

Miss H.: Well, it's no surprise my clothes are much too big.

Nurse: **I'm going to refer you to the dietician and ask her to come and do a full nutritional assessment and see how we can provide you with enough nutrients and fluid while we wait for all the tests [investigations] to be done. Meanwhile, we can order things like scrambled eggs, and give you soup and drinks with added nutrients [fortified] if you're sure that won't make you sick.**

Miss H.: I'm sure that will be fine, thank you.

Case history – Mr Wakefield

Mr Wakefield is a farmer. His son Tom also works on the farm and lives with his wife and two children in the main farmhouse. Mr Wakefield moved to a smaller house on the farm when his wife died about 6 months ago. The last 6 months have been very difficult for Mr Wakefield, and he has come into the health centre to see the practice nurse about feeling generally unwell.

Nurse: Hello Mr Wakefield. How are you today?

Mr W.: Not up to much [a term used to describe feeling generally unwell or having a low mood]. You know – it's hard to feel interested in anything these days.

Nurse: Yes, it must be about 6 months since your wife died.

Mr W.: It will be exactly 6 months on Wednesday. Her dying like that really hit me for six [dealt a severe blow or disappointment]. Tom does his best, but I miss her so much. I can't keep on like this [can't continue in this condition].

Nurse: What do you mean?

Mr W.: I can't leave Tom to run [manage] everything, but I feel dreadful [an emotional phrase to express feeling very unwell].

Nurse: In what way do you feel unwell?

Mr W.: Most of it's my own fault. I know it's bad for me.

Nurse: Bad for you?

Mr W.: The evenings are so long without her [his wife] and at first I thought a couple of drinks [meaning alcoholic drinks] would help me unwind [relax] and get through until bedtime.

Nurse: Did it help?

Mr W.: Not really and I ended up having more than a couple of drinks.

Nurse: Many more?

Mr W.: Oh yes, most evenings I manage a bottle of wine and some whisky, and then regret it in the morning.

Nurse: How do you feel in the morning?

Mr W.: Headache and generally lousy [unwell]. I can't face breakfast and I'm often sick [vomit].

Nurse: Do you take anything for the headache?

Mr W.: A couple of aspirin, but they give me terrible [severe] indigestion.

Nurse: **You have obviously been thinking about the amount of alcohol you drink.**

Mr W.: Yes, it's worrying me. What if I can't stop and become an alcoholic or something?

Nurse: **How much do you think you're having in a week?**

Mr W.: I know that there are sensible limits in units, but I don't know what they are.

Nurse: **Most men can safely drink 3–4 units a day without a significant risk. A unit is 10 grams of alcohol and this is half a pint [an Imperial measure, see Ch. 11] of standard strength beer or one glass of wine or one pub measure of spirits. Some stronger wines have more than 1 unit. The recommended level is 21–28 units for a man spread over 1 week. It's best to avoid binge drinking [uncontrolled drinking] and keep 1 or 2 days when you don't drink.**

Mr W.: My intake is well over the sensible limit. Most nights I probably have over 10 units. I need to do something about it.

Nurse: **You seem to have made up your mind to reduce your intake of alcohol. Have you thought about how you might do this?**

Mr W.: I don't want to give up [stop] drinking completely. In the past I enjoyed a drink in moderation and that's what I want to aim for. Some people say that they never touch a drop [in this case never drink alcohol], but that's not for me.

Nurse: **It's good to have a realistic goal, and drinking in moderation may have health benefits, such as reducing heart disease.**

Mr W.: All this booze [slang for alcohol] has made me put on weight [weight increased], so it will be healthier if I cut down [reduce] on drinking and lose weight.

Nurse: **Are evenings the only time that you have a drink?**

Mr W.: Yes, when I'm on my own [alone].

Nurse: **What can you do to change the pattern?**

Mr W.:   I used to enjoy a walk round the farm of an evening and my grandsons keep badgering [pestering] me to take them out.

Nurse: **Do you think that's possible?**

Mr W.:   Yes, and I think it would help.

Nurse: **I would like to see how you get on [check on your progress]. Perhaps we can make another appointment, and while you're here we can make you an appointment with Doctor Welch. She can arrange for support from a counsellor, and she might think that you would benefit from some medication.**

Mr W.:   Yes, I know I need some proper help and it's such a relief to have told someone about my drinking. I could never tell Tom. It would cause too much bother [upset].

ELIMINATION

Some nursing/medical or Standard English words and corresponding colloquial words and expressions associated with elimination are given in Box 5.6.

Note: Colloquial expressions used in the case histories and example conversations are explained in brackets […].

Case history – Mrs Carter

Mrs Carter has been admitted to the coronary care unit for treatment of unstable angina. She has had angina for about 2 years. During a conversation about the need to use a commode by the bed in order to reduce exertion and hence the oxygen needed by the heart muscle [myocardium], she tells you that she has trouble with her waterworks [urinary tract, especially the bladder].

Nurse: **What sort of problem with your waterworks?**

Mrs C.:   I can't hold on and I leak urine [incontinent of urine]. It's so embarrassing.

Nurse: **It sounds like you have two separate problems.**

Box 5.6 Words associated with elimination (for further examples see Ch. 6)

Nursing/medical or Standard English words	Colloquial (everyday) or slang (very informal) words and expressions used by patients
Constipation	Bunged up; clogged up; costive; haven't been for days; not going properly
Defaecate	Go to the toilet; have bowels open; do number two; pass a motion or stool; to do one's business; to have a clear out
Diarrhoea	Gippy tummy; loose motion; runs; squitters; to be taken short; trots
Faeces; stool	Business; motion; number two; pooh
Flatulence	Belching; feel bloated; gas; wind
Incontinence	Have an accident; I leak; leaky; messed myself; not able to hold on; wet myself
Micturition/urinate	Number one; go to the loo/toilet; pass water; pass urine, pee; spend a penny; tiddle; wee or wee-wee
Lavatory	Bathroom; bog; cloakroom; convenience; gents'; ladies'; latrine; lav.; little girls' room; loo; privy; smallest room; toilet; washroom; water closet (WC)
Urine	Pee; water
Urinary tract	Waterworks (especially the bladder)

Mrs C.: I hadn't thought of it as two problems, but it does happen at different times. The main problem is the need to pass water [micturate] so often and when I need the toilet [lavatory] it is all of a rush [urgent]. Sometimes I don't make it in time and wet myself [incontinent of urine]. The leaking happens when I cough or laugh.

Nurse: How often do you pass water [micturate]?

Mrs C.: Every couple [two] of hours or so [approximately] during the day.

Nurse: What about at night, do you have to get up in the night [to pass water]?

Mrs C.: Oh yes, I have to keep getting up [frequently get out of bed to urinate]. Always twice a night and sometimes more often.

Nurse: When did you start having problems?

Mrs C.: Just after I retired. I'm 68 now, so it must be about 4 years ago.

Nurse: Have you told your GP or the practice nurse?

Mrs C.: I felt too embarrassed and it's something that happens when you get older isn't it? It really limits my social life and it worries me that I might smell.

Nurse: It is more common in older people, but there are different causes and many can be successfully treated. How do you normally cope with the problem?

Mrs C.: I try to be near a toilet, but that's not always easy if I'm out. There are not many public toilets and some of them are not very clean. I wear a sanitary towel [normally used during menstruation] in my knickers [pants, underwear] to cope with the leaks, but I still have plenty of washing to do [implying that this does not always work].

Nurse: I will add all this to your care plan and make sure that everyone knows to bring the commode as soon as you ask. Would you like a supply of towels and disposal bags to keep in the locker?

Mrs C.: Yes please.

Nurse: When your angina has settled down and you are feeling better I will arrange for the continence nurse specialist to come to see you. She is the expert and will be able to do a full assessment and suggest ways of improving the situation.

Mrs C.: I wish I'd told someone earlier, but I thought that you had to grin and bear it [put up with it]. I had no idea that anything could be done.

Nurse: While we're waiting I'd like to have a specimen [sample] of your water to test, and if that shows that you might have an infection we can collect a midstream specimen of urine for the laboratory.

Mrs C.: Is that the test where you have to pee [micturate] into a pot?

Nurse: Yes, that's the one, but we only need the middle bit of the flow, not the urine that comes out first. Have you noticed any blood in your urine or an unusual smell?

Mrs C.: No, nothing like that.

Nurse: What about pain when you pass urine? Does it burn or sting?

Mrs C.: No, I had cystitis when I was younger and I know how painful it is when you go [when she passes urine; micturates].

Nurse: We also need to know how often you are passing urine and how much fluid you are having, but as we are already recording fluid balance for you we will have that information.

Mrs C.: You will tell the nurses about how urgent it is when I ask for the commode?

Nurse: Don't worry I'm putting it on the care plan now, and I will tell the nurse who takes over from me tonight. Do you think you could give me that sample now?

Mrs C.: Yes.

Nurse: Have you any questions before I go and get the commode?

Mrs C.: No, I'm looking forward to feeling better and seeing the specialist nurse about the waterworks.

Case history – Mr Norton

Mr Norton fractured his femur in a motorcycle accident 2 weeks ago. The fracture is being managed with skeletal traction and

Mr Norton has accepted that he will be much less active than usual and will be in hospital for some weeks. He had started to feel better after the accident and the pain in his leg was gradually subsiding, but now he feels bloated [blown up, distended], lethargic and has no appetite.

Mr N.:   I feel terrible [very bad], really out of sorts [unwell].

Nurse: **What's the trouble?**

Mr N.:   I haven't been properly for days [has not defaecated properly for days and is constipated].

Nurse: **When did you last have your bowels open [defaecate]?**

Mr N.:   Saturday was OK, so that's 4 days ago. I wish I'd said earlier, but it seemed stupid to be worried about not going [defaecating] when I'm laid-up [confined to bed] with a leg that's broke [fractured].

Nurse: **How often do you usually go?**

Mr N.:   Every day without fail.

Nurse: **It's probably happened because you're not as active as usual and having to use a bedpan doesn't help.**

Mr N.:   Well I can't do much with the traction and stuff.

Nurse: **How is it making you feel?**

Mr N.:   I'm all blown up and full of wind [flatulence]. Look at my stomach [abdomen], it's huge. I couldn't eat nothing and my mum [mother] had brought in a Chinese [a takeaway meal] as a treat.

Nurse: **Yes, your abdomen is a bit distended. Have you any pain?**

Mr N.:   A bit. It feels like colic [usually refers to intermittent abdominal pain, most often from the intestine, but sometimes from other structures].

Nurse: **What was your motion [faeces; stool] like on Saturday?**

Mr N.:   Just a few hard bits and I had to strain [push hard] to get that out.

Nurse: **What it's like normally?**

Mr N.:   Normal – soft and not having to strain. Except when I've got the runs [diarrhoea] after too much beer and a curry.

Nurse: Was there any pain passing the hard motion, or blood when you cleaned yourself?

Mr N.:   No pain and I didn't see no blood. If I had I would have said straight away [immediately, at once].

Nurse: Did you feel that you hadn't passed a complete motion?

Mr N.:   Yeah [yes], my back passage [rectum] felt full just as if there was more to come.

Nurse: I'll get Dr Cox to write you up for [prescribe] some medicine [laxative] to make you go and we can ask the physio. [short for 'physiotherapist'] to suggest some exercises to help.

Mr N.:   My gran [grandmother] swears by [relies on] her bottle of bowel medicine.

Nurse: You might need some suppositories or a micro enema to get things started and then a few doses of an oral laxative. Hopefully you won't need a whole bottle. It will also help if you can drink more water and choose food high in fibre from the menu.

Mr N.:   Yeah alright, but I don't want salad every meal.

PERSONAL CARE – CLEANSING AND DRESSING, SKIN CARE

Some nursing/medical or Standard English words and correspon-ding colloquial words and expressions associated with personal care are given in Box 5.7.

Note: Colloquial expressions used in the case histories and example conversations are explained in brackets [...].

Case history – Mrs McBride

Mrs McBride lives alone, and Sue her daughter-in-law [the wife of Mrs McBride's son] pops in [visits] most days to take her a meal and check that she is all right. Recently, Sue has noticed that Mrs McBride is increasingly frail and takes a long time to answer the door or make a drink.

Nurse: Hello Mrs McBride. I'm Nurse Ramos. I think you are expecting me. I've come in to see how you are managing at home.

Mrs M.:   Hello dear [an endearment often used by older people] come in. Yes, I knew you were coming. Sue mentioned it earlier when she was in with my lunch [meal in the middle of the day]. She's a good girl to me.

Nurse: I've got a checklist to complete, but it's usually better if you tell me in your own words how you think you are managing. What about if we start with any difficulties you might be having with washing and dressing?

Box 5.7   Words associated with personal care (for further examples see Ch. 6)

Nursing/medical or Standard English words	Colloquial (everyday) or slang (very informal) words and expressions used by patients
Bath/bathe	Have a soak; scrub down
Contusion	Bruise
Dandruff	Scurf
Emollient	Moisturiser
Erythema	Redness
Excoriation	Soreness
Halitosis	Bad breath; mouth odour
Oral hygiene	Brush/clean teeth; mouth wash
Pressure ulcer	Bedsore; pressure sore
Pruritus	Itching (intense)
Rash	Spots/spotty
Wash	Hair wash; hands and face wash; strip wash; wash at the sink/basin

Mrs M.: Yes, that's fine. I've always been as fit as a fiddle [in very good health], but since the winter it's got more and more difficult. Well I am 83. It's all down to [as a result of] old age I suppose.

Nurse: What's more difficult?

Mrs M.: I struggle a bit with a strip wash [wash all over] at the sink, but I get by [cope]. My feet and back don't get done, and it's hard to stand up to wash down below [genital and perianal area]. I need to hold on to the sink and then I can't soap the flannel.

Nurse: Are you able to have a bath or shower?

Mrs M.: No, I'm not strong enough to get in and out of the bath. I'm frightened of slipping, or getting in and not getting out again.

Nurse: How often did you have a bath when you were able to manage?

Mrs M.: Two or three times a week. Heating the water with the immersion heater costs too much to have a bath every day.

Nurse: How do you heat the water for your strip wash?

Mrs M.: Boil a kettle; I've got one in the bedroom for a cuppa [usually refers to a cup of tea] in the morning. Would you like a cup of tea now?

Nurse: No thanks I had one [cup of tea] just before I came out to see you. Would you like to have a bath if it was possible?

Mrs M.: Oh yes, there's nothing like a soak in the bath for getting clean and relaxing you.

Nurse: I quite agree. Is there anyone who could help you?

Mrs M.: I can't ask Sue. She has three children to get off to school, and I don't want to sit in my dressing gown until she can get here.

Nurse: Would you consider having a bath seat that lowers you into the bath and then goes up when you're ready to get out?

Mrs M.: I'm hopeless with machines. How easy are they to use?

Nurse: Very easy. You have a button to push that lowers and raises the seat. If you like we can arrange for someone from

Social Services to come out and do an assessment. What about washing your hair?

Mrs M.: That's no problem. I can do it at the sink. My neighbour used to be a hairdresser and she comes in every few weeks and gives it a cut and set.

Nurse: **That's handy [convenient].**

Mrs M.: It certainly is. I can't get down the town these days unless Sue takes me. I haven't been shopping on my own for ages [for a long time].

Nurse: **Do you have any problems getting dressed and undressed?**

Mrs M.: Some things take for ever [a long time], like putting on tights or trousers.

Nurse: **What about doing things up – buttons and zips, etc.?**

Mrs M.: I make sure that clothes do up at the front – no good struggling with a zip at the back of a dress.

Nurse: **The occupational therapist can suggest some simple gadgets [appliances, devices] to help with dressing and show you about easier ways of doing things. Would you like me to arrange for her to come?**

Mrs M.: Yes please. Another neighbour, Mrs Smith at number 80 [the house number], had a visit from one of them and she got on very well.

Case history – Mr Dafnis

Mr Dafnis is going to have planned [elective] surgery. He has a long history of eczema, with dry, itchy skin. When he attends the pre-admission assessment clinic he expresses some concern about the care of his skin condition while he is in the ward after the major surgical operation.

Mr D.: I'm worried about my eczema when I come into hospital. It's important to follow my usual routine or it will flare up [get worse] again.

Nurse: **How long have you had eczema?**

Mr D.: For years, it's chronic now but some things make it worse.

Nurse: What sort of things?

Mr D.: In my case it's things like getting too hot, such as from the sun shining through a window.

Nurse: We can arrange for you to have a bed well away from any windows. Is there anything else?

Mr D.: Alcohol starts up the itching [pruritus], but I never touch it [does not drink alcohol] nowadays.

Nurse: What's your skin like now?

Mr D.: Not very good. It's very red [erythema] and the itching and scratching is much worse. I put it down to [caused by] the stress of having to have the op. [short for 'operation'].

Nurse: Which areas are worse affected?

Mr D.: Mainly my face, as you can see, and my back is very itchy.

Nurse: Have you any sore areas [excoriation] or weeping [producing exudate] areas?

Mr D.: No, my skin is just dry and very itchy. Any vesicles and broken areas would mean I was open to infection. Is that why you're asking?

Nurse: Yes, exactly. But to be on the safe side I'll get the doctor to have a look now. What measures are you taking to reduce the flare up?

Mr D.: I never use soap because it takes out my natural skin oils, so I use soap substitute, and at the moment I'm using an oily moisturiser [emollient] nearly every hour, but touch wood [a reference to the habit of touching something wooden to avert bad luck] it won't be so bad by the time I come into the ward.

Nurse: Are you using anything other than the emollient on your skin?

Mr D.: No.

Nurse: Have you used steroid ointments lately?

Mr D.: No, not for months. I only have them as a last resort.

Nurse: What about other medicines?

Mr D.: I'm taking an antihistamine so the scratching is reduced and I can get some sleep.

Nurse: I'll make sure that your skin management is written in the care plan. Have you any questions?

Mr D.: What if my eczema gets really bad before I'm due to come in?

Nurse: If it gets any worse please let us know. I'll be giving you some printed information with the unit telephone number in any case.

Mr D.: OK, thanks.

SLEEPING

Some nursing/medical or Standard English words and corresponding colloquial words and expressions associated with sleeping are given in Box 5.8.

Note: Colloquial expressions used in the case histories and example conversations are explained in brackets [...].

Case history – Mrs Bell

Mrs Bell moved into the care home from sheltered housing [housing with communal areas and a warden] 5 days ago. She had enjoyed her time there, but after the fall and the fractured hip she felt that she needed more care. Although there was a button to press to get help, she was frightened of falling again and having to wait for help to come. Both her sons were concerned about her and going into the home seemed the most sensible thing to do. She hadn't expected to feel at home straight away, but she is missing her friends and is not sleeping well.

Nurse: Good morning Mrs Bell how are you settling in?

Mrs B.: Not too bad I suppose, but it feels a bit strange still.

Nurse: I thought it would be helpful for us to have a chat now that you have been here for a few days. You said that it feels strange.

Mrs B.: I'm not complaining and everyone is so kind, but I miss the ladies from the sheltered housing.

Nurse: Have any of them visited you yet?

Box 5.8 Words associated with sleeping (for further examples see Ch. 6)	
Nursing/medical or Standard English words	Colloquial (everyday) or slang (very informal) words and expressions used by patients
Bruxism	Grind my teeth during sleep
Go to bed/sleep	Hit the hay/sack; retire for the night; say goodnight; turn in
Insomnia	Awake half the night; can't get off (to sleep); sleeplessness; wakefulness; wide awake
Narcolepsy	Drop off without warning
Sleep	Catnap; doze/dozing off; drop off; forty winks; kip; lose myself; nap; siesta; shut eye; snooze
Sleep hygiene	Bed time or pre-sleep routine/rituals
Somnambulance	Sleep walking
Somnolent	Dozy; drowsy; heavy-eyed; nodding off; sleepy
Weary	Dead beat; dog-tired; done in; ready to drop; whacked

Mrs B.: The warden came yesterday and it was nice to hear all the gossip. My special friends are away on their hols [holiday] until next week, so I expect they will be round then.

Nurse: That's good. What about your sons?

Mrs B.: John brought me in, and he came yesterday on his way home from work. Nigel works away during the week, but he will be in on Saturday.

Nurse: Have you got to know the other residents yet?

Mrs B.: I had tea [a light meal in the afternoon or evening] with Mrs Forbes and she was very friendly.

Nurse: How are you sleeping?

Mrs B.: Not very well, I'm awake half the night.

Nurse: Is that usual for you?

Mrs B.: Not really. I used to have the odd [in this context means 'infrequent' or 'unusual'] night when I would wake up, but most nights I would sleep right through until about half past six [6.30 a.m.].

Nurse: Do you have trouble falling asleep [going to sleep] or do you wake up in the night?

Mrs B.: I'm really tired, but as soon as I put the light out I'm wide awake again.

Nurse: Do you get to sleep eventually?

Mrs B.: Yes, but then I wake up feeling whacked [weary] and groggy [unwell]. I don't feel rested.

Nurse: Do you wake up earlier than usual?

Mrs B.: I did this morning. There was a lot of coming and going [activity] because the lady in the next room was poorly [unwell].

Nurse: Yes, she had to go into hospital.

Mrs B.: And I'm so tired in the day I keep dozing off [going to sleep] in the chair.

Nurse: Did you usually have a short nap [sleep] during the day before you came to us?

Mrs B.: Well, if I'm honest, I did sometimes put my feet up [relax] after the lunchtime Archers [a long-running radio programme] and lose myself for a bit [have a short sleep].

Nurse: What time have you been falling asleep in the chair?

Mrs B.: After supper [last meal of the day], so when I come to [wake up] it's time to start thinking about going to bed. That's a bit late for a nap I know.

Nurse: Do you have a bedtime routine – things that help you get to sleep?

Mrs B.: I used to have a bath last thing [just before going to bed] and take a milky drink to bed. Then read until I felt drowsy [somnolent].

Nurse: What sort of time [approximate timing] would you usually have the bath?

Mrs B.: After the news at ten [10 p.m.] and be in bed by 11 [11 p.m.]. I'm not sure if it's all right to have a bath that late here. I expect the girls [night staff] are too busy to help with baths.

Nurse: I will have a word [discuss it] with the nurse in charge tonight about making sure you can have a bath if you want, and get a milky drink. It is so important to get a good night's sleep.

Mrs B.: You can say that again [emphasises the importance of the nurse's last statement]. I would be very grateful if they could help me with a bath.

Nurse: Is there anything else that can be done to help you sleep properly?

Mrs B.: It is quite warm in my room. I'm not used to having the radiator so hot in the bedroom.

Nurse: We can turn the thermostat down, so it just takes the chill off the room [make sure that the room is not cold].

Mrs B.: They tried last night, but it was too stiff to turn.

Nurse: I'll get on to [contact] the maintenance staff right away [at once].

Mrs B.: It was so hot I pushed the duvet off me. I haven't done that since the change [climacteric/menopause] when I used to have night sweats.

Nurse: What about when you get up in the morning, will you be warm enough?

Mrs B.: Oh yes, my boys [her sons] treated me to [paid for] some new clothes to come in here and that included a fleecy dressing gown. Look it's on the chair. Do you think it's too bright?

Nurse: I like that dark pink. It's such a warm colour.

Mrs B.: Yes, I like it. I did wonder about pink at my age, but then I thought 'Why not?'.

Nurse: Is there anything else that stops you sleeping?

Mrs B.: I still need to get used to [become accustomed to] the light coming in from the corridor.

Nurse: Were you used to sleeping in complete darkness?

Mrs B.: Yes, the sheltered housing is on the edge of the village, right out in the sticks [rural location, in the countryside].

Nurse: **We need to keep the light on in the corridor, so that everyone can move about safely.**

Mrs B.: Yes, I know. I don't suppose it will bother [trouble] me for long.

WORKING AND PLAYING

Some nursing/medical or Standard English words and corresponding colloquial words and expressions associated with working and playing are given in Box 5.9.

Note: Colloquial expressions used in the case histories and example conversations are explained in brackets […].

Case history – Mr Khan

Mr Khan is about to be discharged home after having a myocardial infarction a week ago. He normally helps to run the family business and needs to drive all over the UK to see customers. He is anxious about how a recent myocardial infarction will affect his driving, the business and his leisure activities.

Mr K.: Nurse Brown, have you got a minute [the time] to talk?

Nurse: **I need to give a painkiller to another patient. I'll be back in 5 minutes.**

Mr K.: OK.

Nurse: **Right, Mr Khan I'm back. What would you like to talk about?**

Mr K.: I'm really worried about how I'll manage to run my part of the business after the heart attack [myocardial infarction].

Nurse: **Did you speak to the cardiac nurse specialist?**

Mr K.: Yes, on Tuesday. She explained everything and I asked lots of questions. It all seemed quite straightforward [easy, simple], but now that I'm dressed and ready to go home I'm not so sure.

Box 5.9 Words associated with working and playing (for further examples see Ch. 6)

Nursing/medical or Standard English words	Colloquial (everyday) or slang (very informal) words and expressions used by patients
Dismissed	Fired; given my cards; given the boot; given my notice; given the push; got the sack; laid off; let go; marching orders; sacked; sent packing
Employed	Hired; in a job; in work; paid work; working
Employee	Bread-winner; wage-earner; worker
Employer	Boss; gaffer; governor
Leisure/leisure activities	Amusement; breathing space; free time; fun; hobby; pastime; play; pleasure; recreation; R&R; spare time; time off
Occupation; profession	Business; career; calling (outdated); craft; job; line of work; livelihood; position; trade; walk of life; work
Relaxation	Chill out; laze about; let one's hair down; loosen up; put one's feet up; take it easy; unwind
Retired	Given up work; pensioner; pensioned off; put out to grass
Self-employed	Freelance; my own boss; work for myself
Unemployed	Jobless; looking for a job/work; not working; on the dole/social; out of work

Nurse: Did she leave the printed information?

Mr K.: Yes.

Nurse: What bits are worrying you?

Mr K.: Well, mainly the driving and getting back to work. I drive about 20 000 miles a year on business. There is something in the leaflet about driving, but I'm worried that Swansea [the location of the Driver and Vehicle

Licensing Agency (DVLA); the word 'Swansea' may be used to describe it in conversation] will take my licence away.

Nurse: **Is yours an ordinary licence?**

Mr K.: I should think so.

Nurse: **You don't drive a bus or a lorry do you?**

Mr K.: No, just the car and sometimes the minibus for the Community Centre.

Nurse: **You will need to stop driving for at least 4 weeks and you don't have to notify DVLA. You have an appointment to see Dr Bradley [the cardiologist] next month. He will advise you about when you can start driving again.**

Mr K.: I hope it's not much longer than 4 weeks. My dad [father] and brother can visit the customers for a few weeks, but not for ever.

Nurse: **So far your recovery has gone well. There's no reason to think you won't be fit [well enough] to drive in a month. It might be a good idea to tell your insurance company about the heart attack.**

Mr K.: Yes, that's sensible. I don't want to drive without insurance. That means a fine and six points on your licence.

Nurse: **You mentioned getting back to work.**

Mr K.: We run a small family business, so one person off sick puts a real strain on everyone else.

Nurse: **Yes, I can see that. Do you do most of the customer visiting?**

Mr K.: Yes, my dad doesn't really like driving long distances and my brother is better at the day-to-day business.

Nurse: **Again Dr Bradley will advise you about going back to work, but most people gradually increase their activity and are back at work in 4–6 weeks. It would be longer if you had a job with a lot of physical activity.**

Mr K.: No, if I'm in the office it's mainly computer work and telephoning customers. My job isn't very active, but I'm keen on sport.

Nurse:	What sport do you do?
Mr K.:	I play some cricket and coach some lads [boys, youngsters] in a local football team.
Nurse:	How active is the coaching?
Mr K.:	Well I work-out [train] with the boys. I'm keen to keep on [continue] with both the cricket and the coaching.
Nurse:	The staff running [organising] the formal sessions of the cardiac rehabilitation programme will be able to give you information about safe levels of exercise and playing sport. When do you start?
Mr K.:	The specialist nurse said that she will give me a ring [telephone] next week to see how we're getting on [coping] at home and by then she will know the dates for the exercise sessions.
Nurse:	Don't forget the cardiac nurses have a telephone helpline if you have any worries once you get home, and you can also use their e-mail.
Mr K.:	Yes, it's very reassuring to know that there is some back-up [support].
Nurse:	Have you any questions about your drugs and the dietary changes, or anything else?
Mr K.:	No, that's all the worries for now. I just needed to get those things straight [sorted] in my mind.

Case history – Mrs Hamilton

Mrs Hamilton has had diabetes for many years and her vision is deteriorating due to diabetic retinopathy. She and her husband are both retired and enjoy walking and gardening.

Nurse:	Hello Mrs Hamilton. It doesn't seem like a year since we last saw you.
Mrs H.:	Yes, time for the annual eye check again.
Nurse:	Not everyone is so reliable about attending as you.
Mrs H.:	I'd be daft [foolish, unwise] not to. Finding problems early is so important. My sight is already bad, I don't want it to get any worse.

Nurse: I will be putting the eye drops in to dilate your pupil, so we can examine the back of your eye [retina]. How has your sight been since last year's check?

Mrs H.:   I'm finding it more difficult to read small print and I've got patchy [uneven] blurring of vision. It does make life difficult.

Nurse: How does it affect you on a day-to-day basis?

Mrs H.:   Now Jim [her husband] and I have given up working [retired] we have time to do our garden. I have always had green fingers [keen gardener] and we like walking in the countryside, but it's not much fun with my poor vision. I have to rely on Jim to read the labels on weed killer for the garden and the plant labels at the garden centre. He doesn't mind, but I mind very much. I feel so helpless and frustrated about losing my independence.

Nurse: Yes, it must be frustrating.

Mrs H.:   I'm really cheesed off [fed up]. It's reading books as well. I like to relax with a book after supper [last meal of the day] while Jim has a pint [in this context it means beer] at our local [nearest public house]. But now I can only see if the print is very large and every light in the room is on. It's not very relaxing.

Nurse: No, it doesn't sound very relaxing. Have you got any low vision aids?

Mrs H.:   I've got my glasses [spectacles] and a magnifier and I make sure that the lighting is right for what I'm doing.

Nurse: How is your diabetic control?

Mrs H.:   OK. I'm doing quite well with the sugar control and the insulin injections are no problem now I use a preloaded insulin pen [device for injecting insulin].

Nurse: I'm sure you know how important this is to help stop the retinopathy from getting worse.

Mrs H.:   Oh yes, the diabetic nurse specialists are always harping on about [emphasising] the importance of managing the diabetes properly.

Nurse: We all nag [keep on at] you, don't we?

Mrs H.:   I don't mind. But just think, if I hadn't gone after [applied for] the area manager post [job] and had to have a medical [routine health check] it might have been ages [long time] before they found the diabetes and I started the insulin and a proper diet.

SEXUALITY

Some nursing/medical or Standard English words and corresponding colloquial words and expressions associated with sexuality are given in Box 5.10.

Note: Colloquial expressions used in the case histories and example conversations are explained in brackets [...].

Box 5.10 Words associated with sexuality (for further examples see Ch. 6)	
Nursing/medical or Standard English words	Colloquial (everyday) or slang (very informal) words and expressions used by patients
Cervix	Neck of womb
Dysmenorrhoea	Painful periods
Erectile dysfunction	Impotent
Genitalia	Bits; down below; down there, naughty bits; private parts; privates
Menorrhagia	Flooding; heavy periods
Menstruation	Being unwell; having the curse, period(s)
Sexual intercourse	Go to bed with; intimacy; lovemaking; make love; sex; sexual relations; sleep with; to do/have it
Uterus	Womb

Case history – Mr Johns

Mr Johns has been a widower [a man whose wife has died and has not remarried] for many years. He is generally fit [in good health], apart from hypertension which is treated with enalapril maleate.

Mr J.:   I've been under the doctor [in the doctor's care, being treated] for my blood pressure. She said to make an appointment for you to check me over and do the blood pressure.

Nurse: **What has the doctor prescribed?**

Mr J.:   Innovace [proprietary name for enalapril maleate].

Nurse: **How have you been?**

Mr J.:   Not bad [In English, when you have two negatives, known as a 'double negative', it creates a middle way, meaning not a positive ('very good'), but not a negative ('very bad') either].

Nurse: **What, not feeling really well?**

Mr J.:   A bit seedy [unwell], but nothing specific.

Nurse: **Is there anything worrying you?**

Mr J.:   I've met a nice lady, we really hit it off [get on well]. She likes all the same things as me, music, food and everything.

Nurse: **Had you been on your own for long?**

Mr J.:   A long time. Jenny [his wife] died of cancer 10 years ago. I didn't want anyone else at first, but when the kids [children] married and moved away I felt a bit lonely and that.

Nurse: **Yes.**

Mr J.:   I met someone at work, but that soon fizzled out [came to nothing].

Nurse: **Some men can have difficulty with erections when taking the medicine you are on. Have you had any trouble?**

Mr J.:   It's difficult to talk about it, but I was impotent [had erectile dysfunction] and couldn't do it [have sexual intercourse]. I told myself it was just nerves being with someone new and tiredness.

Nurse: Yes, it's difficult to talk about intimate things.

Mr J.: I'm worried about my new relationship. I don't want anything to go wrong like last time.

Nurse: We're lucky in this area to have a nurse who specialises in the management of erectile dysfunction, that's the medical term for problems with erections. Would you like me to arrange an assessment appointment with him?

Mr J.: Yes please, I need to talk to someone. When the doctor gave me the script [short for prescription] she said one of the side-effects was trouble with erections, but how could I ask her any questions? It was so embarrassing.

Case history – Mrs Hall

Problems with menstruation have been part of Mrs Hall's life for as long as she can remember. First it was dysmenorrhoea as a teenager and into her 20s, and now 20 years later she has menorrhagia and the dysmenorrhoea is back. She has seen the consultant and the plan is for her to come in as a day case for a hysteroscopy and endometrial biopsy.

Nurse: Hello again Mrs Hall. I've come to answer any questions you might have about having the examination as a day case.

Mrs H.: You and the consultant explained that he would look inside the womb [uterus] with a special instrument and then do a scrape [dilatation and curettage] to get a sample for testing, so I'm fairly clear about what will happen.

Nurse: Have you any questions about the possible complications of the procedure?

Mrs H.: No, I'm fully aware that there is a risk of the womb being perforated.

Nurse: You signed your consent form and consented to a general anaesthetic.

Mrs H.: I didn't fancy [like the idea of] having it done in outpatients, I'd rather be put to sleep [anaesthetised] first.

Nurse: It will only be a short anaesthetic. You should be able to go home later that afternoon/evening. Will your partner be collecting you?

Mrs H.: Yes, he'll come straight from work. His shift finishes at 3 o'clock, so it will be about 4 [4.00 p.m.]. Is that OK?

Nurse: No problem, but he should ring [telephone] first just to see if you are recovered enough to go home. You might still be a bit sleepy.

Mrs H.: Mr Bainbridge said you could give me a date for the examination.

Nurse: Yes, I'll get the dates up on the computer, but first I need to check a few things with you.

Mrs H.: OK.

Nurse: We do the examinations on a Wednesday morning. Are there any dates that we need to avoid?

Mrs H.: No, we're not going away [in this context means away on holiday] until the problems with my periods [menstruation] have been sorted out.

Nurse: We will need to avoid dates when you have your period, as it makes it difficult to get a good view of the inside of the womb. Are your periods regular?

Mrs H.: Fairly. It usually comes every 30 days or so. The real problem is that it lasts much longer.

Nurse: How long?

Mrs H.: The last 3 months have been dreadful, with the heavy bleeding going on for 7 or 8 days.

Nurse: Does that make things difficult for you?

Mrs H.: Yes, very difficult, because I keep flooding [excessive bleeding from the uterus]. Sometimes the blood comes through the pad and my clothes, so I'm scared [frightened] to go out. Plus I'm forever washing clothes and the bedding.

Nurse: It sounds as if your daily activities are seriously affected.

Mrs H.: Yes, they are. I can't plan to do anything for a whole week every month.

Nurse: Do you have any spotting [intermenstrual bleeding], such as after having sexual intercourse?

Mrs H.: No, only the heavy bleeding [menorrhagia] and flooding during my period. But it's affecting our sex life; either I'm bleeding or too tired.

Nurse: The blood test we took will show if you are anaemic. Heavy periods often cause anaemia and that would make you tired.

Mrs H.: I really want the bleeding sorted. It's really dragging me down [making me ill, emotionally and physically].

Nurse: The examination will help to find a physical cause, but as you know Mr Bainbridge thinks that you may have dysfunctional uterine bleeding and he might not find a physical cause.

Mrs H.: I'm in agony [in extreme pain] with period pains [dysmenorrhoea] as well. I used to have pain with my periods when I was young, but this pain is much worse.

Nurse: What do you take for it?

Mrs H.: Just paracetamol, but they don't do much good [not very effective]. I know I said that I want it sorted, but I'm worried in case he says I need a hysterectomy.

Nurse: There are several different treatments for heavy bleeding, such as tablets, hormones and a fairly new technique called ablation, where the lining of the womb is removed. There is lots to try before hysterectomy needs to be considered.

Mrs H.: I do hope so. You hear about women having a hysterectomy and never really getting over it [recovering], plus all those things that happen to you.

Nurse: What sort of things?

Mrs H.: Well you put on weight.

Nurse: There is no reason for anyone to put on weight after a hysterectomy other than the usual reasons of eating too much and not getting enough exercise.

Mrs H.: It wouldn't feel right somehow.

Nurse: **In what way?**

Mrs H.: You know – not feeling like a proper woman.

Nurse: **If Mr Bainbridge advised a hysterectomy and you were considering it, the usual thing would be for you to see one of us specialist nurses again to have a proper discussion about the operation before it went ahead. But we could talk it through [discuss fully] now if you would like to.**

Mrs H.: Yes please, if you've got time now.

ANXIETY, STRESS AND DEPRESSION

Some nursing/medical or Standard English words and corresponding colloquial words and expressions associated with anxiety, stress and depression are given in Box 5.11.

Box 5.11 Words associated with anxiety, stress and depression (for further examples see Ch. 6)	
Nursing/medical or Standard English words	Colloquial (everyday) or slang (very informal) words and expressions used by patients
Anxious	Jumpy; nervy; wired (often used in connection with substance misuse)
Depressed	Down in the dumps/mouth; feeling down; got the hump; hacked or naffed off (also means annoyed); low (*Note:* Many of these expressions describe mild mood change rather than a depressive illness)
Mental health problem	Barmy; batty; bonkers; cracked/crackers; crazy; cuckoo; loony; loopy; mad; mental; nuts/nutty; off one's chump/head/rocker/trolley; out of one's mind; round the bend; screw loose; screwy
Stressed	Strung out; up tight

Note: Colloquial expressions used in the case histories and example conversations are explained in brackets [...].

Case history – Mr Reeves

Mr Reeves has always worried about things at work and often becomes anxious if he can't clear his desk each day. Recently, he doesn't seem to be able to concentrate properly and has been staying late at work to get the day's jobs finished. He has started to feel anxious about returning to work after the weekend, and on two occasions he has had a panic attack during the bus ride to work on a Monday morning.

Nurse: Hello Mr Reeves. I'm Nurse Owen. Is it all right if I ask you some questions?

Mr R.: Yes.

Nurse: I understand that you have had some panic attacks.

Mr R.: Yes, when I had to go back to work after the weekend.

Nurse: Tell me what happened.

Mr R.: It came out of the blue [suddenly, without warning]. I felt uneasy and came over [felt] all sweaty, my heart was pounding [palpitations] and my chest felt like it would burst. I thought I was about to snuff it [die].

Nurse: What did you do?

Mr R.: I tried to calm down and take some big breaths, but it didn't work [not effective] and I had to get off the bus in a hurry and pushed my way off. People must have thought I was round the bend [have a mental health problem].

Nurse: Did you get to work in the end?

Mr R.: No, I needed to get home.

Nurse: Were things any better once you got home?

Mr R.: The panic had gone, but I felt edgy [nervous, irritable].

Nurse: How do you mean?

Mr R.: I couldn't settle to anything [moved from task to task] and was fidgety [nervously touching or playing with things] all day.

Nurse:	Tell me about your job.
Mr R.:	I work for an insurance company in the claims department.
Nurse:	**What does that involve?**
Mr R.:	I deal with claims from clients. It's mainly people damaging things at home or perhaps they have had a break-in [burglary]. It must be dreadful and I worry about getting the claims agreed quickly if someone has had a break-in.
Nurse:	**Do your managers put pressure on you to complete claims within a set time?**
Mr R.:	Yes, it's all about targets and outcomes, but you must know. It's like that in the NHS these days.
Nurse:	**Yes, most people seem to have pressures at work.**
Mr R.:	It started when I wanted be the quickest to get claims sorted out.
Nurse:	**What happened?**
Mr R.:	I was working against the clock [pushed for time] and I managed for a while, but then I felt that I must complete everything the same day.
Nurse:	**Was that realistic?**
Mr R.:	No, but I couldn't see that. I stayed most evenings, but seemed to get less and less done.
Nurse:	**Why do you think that happened?**
Mr R.:	I couldn't concentrate and went from job to job without finishing it. I couldn't deal with claims that were anything out of the ordinary [unusual].
Nurse:	**How did you cope?**
Mr R.:	Well I didn't cope. I just put them to the bottom of my pile of work.
Nurse:	**How has the work situation affected your daily life?**
Mr R.:	I'm finding it hard to get out of the house [leave] for work in the mornings.
Nurse:	**Anything else?**
Mr R.:	Same sort of problems as the ones at work. I can't concentrate on one thing and keep starting things and

then leaving it to start something else. Doing the shopping is a nightmare [in this context means 'an ordeal']. I just wander from aisle to aisle picking items up and putting them down. It takes me over an hour and then I forget lots of items.

Nurse: **Do you feel under stress?**

Mr R.: Most of the time.

Nurse: **What sort of things make you feel stressed?**

Mr R.: Work obviously, but things at home can hassle me [in this context means 'worry'] as well.

Nurse: **At home [in this context reflecting what Mr Reeves has said]?**

Mr R.: Yes, paying bills on time and the state of the garden, it's like a jungle [very untidy]. When I feel uptight [stressed] I get really fussy about piddling [petty, unimportant] things that don't matter.

Nurse: **What do you normally do to relieve the stress?**

Mr R.: Listening to music helps and I've started doing yoga again.

Nurse: **Your GP [general practitioner] thought that our team might be able to offer you some help.**

Mr R.: Yes, we discussed some of the options, but I need more details.

Case history – Mel

Mel, aged 16 years, has just started at a new school. She had to change schools when her parents split up [divorced]. It has been difficult to make new friends and she is worried about the exams in the summer.

Nurse: **Hello, I'm Nurse Sanchez. May I call you Mel?**

Mel: If you like.

Nurse: **What would you like to talk to me about?**

Mel: You know, I moved here last term when my mum [mother] and dad [father] split up [divorced].

Nurse: **Yes, you came from St. Mary's didn't you?**

Mel: Yeah [yes], it was cool [OK, excellent] there.

Nurse: How are you settling in here?

Mel: Don't know really.

Nurse: What about the people in your class? Have you made any friends?

Mel: They've all known each other since year 7 [the first year in high school]. They don't want me – they think I'm stupid.

Nurse: Is that what you think?

Mel: Yeah, 'cos [because] of the row [quarrel] I had with that girl who's always talking.

Nurse: How do you feel about the quarrel?

Mel: It's getting me down [depressing me].

Nurse: Have you felt like crying at all?

Mel: I'm usually OK, as long as [provided] they don't keep picking on [bully, tease] me. During PE [physical education] I burst into tears when they made a thing about not picking me [choosing me] for their team. They said I was naff [in this context means 'useless'] at sport.

Nurse: Do feel like breaking down [bursting into tears] at other times?

Mel: Yeah, sometimes at home for no reason, but my mum [mother] says I should try not to take things to heart [try not to be too hurt by people's remarks].

Nurse: Did you tell your mum that you just felt like crying?

Mel: I don't want to worry her. She's having a bad time.

Nurse: Because of the divorce?

Mel: Yeah, she was gutted [very upset].

Nurse: How have you been feeling generally?

Mel: Sort of sad and fed up [bored, discontented].

Nurse: Are you able to enjoy the things you used to do?

Mel: I can't be bothered to get dolled up [get dressed up]. You can't go out on your own.

Nurse: What about hobbies?

Mel: I used to help out at the local riding stables.

Nurse: Yes?

Mel:	I gave it up [stopped] when we moved to this place. I can't get interested in anything now.
Nurse:	**Apart from what you have told me is there anything else you are particularly worried about?**
Mel:	Yeah, I'm frantic [very worried] about my exams.
Nurse:	**What are you planning to do [career plans, etc.]?**
Mel:	Yeah, I really want to go to uni' [university] to do law, so I need good grades.
Nurse:	**It's difficult changing schools just before exams.**
Mel:	Tell me about it [in this context, emphasises that Mel knows this already].
Nurse:	**How is your studying going?**
Mel:	I should do a plan, but I keep putting it off [delaying]. It's easier to watch TV [television].
Nurse:	**How are you sleeping?**
Mel:	It's difficult to drop off [get to sleep] worrying about my revision.
Nurse:	**What about your appetite?**
Mel:	OK, if you count junk food. If my mum is out I just have chips.
Nurse:	**When you feel sad do you ever feel like harming yourself?**
Mel:	No, not really. I know my mum needs me and I'm set on [determined] being a lawyer.
Nurse:	**Do you think you could talk to your mum about how you're feeling?**
Mel:	I suppose it would be best.
Nurse:	**The doctor might be able to help as well.**
Mel:	Yeah, thanks.

DEMENTIA AND CONFUSION

Some nursing/medical or Standard English words and corresponding colloquial words and expressions associated with dementia and confusion are given in Box 5.12.

Note: Colloquial expressions used in the case histories and example conversations are explained in brackets [...].

Box 5.12 Words associated with dementia and confusion (for further examples see Ch. 6)	
Nursing/medical or Standard English words	Colloquial (everyday) or slang (very informal) words and expressions used by patients
Confused	At a loss; at sea; at sixes and sevens; befuddled; bewildered; mixed up; muddled; muzzy; not with it
Demented	Crack brained; crazed; crazy; daft; dotty; non-compos mentis

Case history – Mrs Georges

Mrs Georges has cared for her husband for over a year. His condition has deteriorated rapidly and he has now been admitted to a nursing home. He has severe dementia due to Alzheimer's disease, and it is impossible for his wife to manage with him at home.

Mrs G.: Hello Nurse. My husband seems quite settled now. Would you like me to answer those questions?

Nurse: Hello. Yes, now's a good time. Tea will be here in half an hour [30 minutes] or so. Will you be staying to have tea with Mr Georges?

Mrs G.: Yes, that would be nice. It's a real treat [pleasure] to sit down and have a meal that someone else has got ready.

Nurse: Being the only carer is such hard work.

Mrs G.: At home he [her husband] wouldn't let me out of his sight for a minute. You can imagine how hard it is to get a meal.

Nurse: Yes, how are you feeling now that Mr Georges is here with us?

Mrs G.: I know it was the right decision and had it all out [discussed it fully] with the people from the Social [social workers], but I'll miss him not being at home.

It had to happen. I'm completely done in [exhausted or worn-out].

Nurse: **Tell me about Mr Georges.**

Mrs G.: I wish you could have seen him before all this happened. He was so on the ball [alert] and always helping people. He was in the merchant navy and spent months away, so I was used to being on my own before he retired.

Nurse: **Have you got family nearby?**

Mrs G.: I won't be lonely. Our lad [son] lives just around the corner. I really lost my Bob [Mr Georges] when his mind started to go.

Nurse: **When did you first notice?**

Mrs G.: Hard to say [difficult], I suppose you expect your memory to get worse, so you put the little lapses down to [caused by] him getting older.

Nurse: **Well we all lose our glasses and forget names.**

Mrs G.: Yes, but it was more than that. He seemed muddled [confused] by everyday things like making a pot of tea. He would put the teabags in the kettle or make the tea with cold water.

Nurse: **How was he in himself?**

Mrs G.: At first he knew something was wrong. He was frustrated and would fly off the handle [be irritable] with me and I would snap back. I didn't realise he couldn't help it [not his fault].

Nurse: **How do you feel about it now?**

Mrs G.: Real bad. I feel weepy [tearful] just talking about it. Silly isn't it?

Nurse: **No it's not silly, not at all.**

Mrs G.: After 40 years married we knew what the other was thinking most of the time and now we're not even on the same wavelength [don't understand one another].

Nurse: **What other things have been happening?**

Mrs G.: He would witter on and on [go on] about the same thing and asking me the same question. I'd say to him

'Bob you're driving me up the wall [irritating me]', he'd smile and next minute do it again. But he hardly says a word now [does not speak very much].

Nurse: **What about washing and dressing?**

Mrs G.: Gets in a right pickle [difficulty] with dressing. I have to help him. It's as if he can't remember what to do. Getting him to shave is a right carry-on [performance], he just won't do it and pushes me away if I try to help. I hate to see him so scruffy [untidy]. He was always so particular with his turn out [clothes and appearance]. I don't know whether you'll have better luck with him.

Nurse: **The care assistants have special training sessions and they're all used to looking after people who have problems like Mr Georges'.**

Mrs G.: But they won't know how to stop him getting in a lather [agitated].

Nurse: **Would you like to meet the team who will be caring for Mr Georges, so you can tell them about the best way to do things? Most relatives say it's reassuring.**

Mrs G.: That would put my mind at rest [feel reassured] about leaving him here. I will just say that he seems to like sitting in front of the box [television]. He can't know what's on but he does seem calmer. Before he got this bad he was forever changing channels and I never got to see the end of anything.

Nurse: **How frustrating for you. Does Mr Georges wander about?**

Mrs G.: In the last few months it started. He kept wandering off during the day. He was off like a shot [moved quickly] and he'd be in the road before I got out the house. I was sure he'd be under a car at any moment [have a road accident]. And then he stopped knowing day and night and would get up [out of bed] at all hours of the night. That really scared me. What if he'd turned on the gas [the gas cooker/oven]? He was always fiddling [touching] with it during the day.

Nurse: **That must have been a real worry.**

Mrs G.: I'd lay there in the dark listening for him getting up, and when I dropped off [got to sleep] any little noise would wake me. That's what really decided me about him coming here.

Nurse: I just heard the tea trolley go by. We can finish this later if you like.

Mrs G.: I could do with a cuppa [usually refers to a cup of tea] I'm parched [thirsty].

PAIN

Some nursing/medical or Standard English words and corresponding colloquial words and expressions associated with pain are given in Box 5.13.

Note: Colloquial expressions used in the case histories and example conversations are explained in brackets [...].

Box 5.13 Words associated with pain (for further examples see Ch. 6)	
Nursing/medical or Standard English words	Colloquial (everyday) or slang (very informal) words and expressions used by patients
Analgesic	Painkiller
Grimaces	Pull a face
Pain	Ache; agony; cramp; discomfort; hurt; irritation; smarting; soreness; spasm; tenderness; throb; twinge (see text for more words used to describe pain)

'Pain' and 'ache' mean the same thing and we speak of 'aches and pains' generally. Both these words are nouns, but the word 'ache' can be used with the following to form a compound noun: backache, earache, headache, stomach-ache (usually means an ache in the abdomen), toothache. For the other parts of the body, we say:

'I have a pain in my shoulder, chest, etc.'

It is possible to have a pain in the back, head and stomach (usually means the abdomen), but this generally refers to a more serious condition than backache, headache and stomach-ache.

The word 'ache' can also be used as a verb:

'My leg aches after walking 10 miles.'

'My back aches after gardening.'

The word 'hurt' is another verb used to express injury and pain:

'My chest hurts when I cough.'

'My neck hurts when I turn my head.'

How patients describe pain: commonly used words

— aching
— beating
— biting
— boring
— burning (as in cystitis, oesophagitis)
— bursting
— colicky (often used to describe the pain that results from periodic spasm in an abdominal organ (biliary, intestinal), but also used to describe renal colic and dysmenorrhoea)
— crampy
— crushing (as in angina pectoris or myocardial infarction)
— cutting (rectal disease)
— discomfort (may describe mild pain sensation)
— dragging (as in uterine prolapse)
— drawing
— dull (headache, tumour)
— gnawing (tumour) (pronounced *nawing*)
— grinding

— griping
— gripping (as in angina pectoris)
— heavy (as pre-menstrual)
— knife-like
— numb (lack of sensation)
— piercing (angina pectoris)
— pinching
— pounding (headache – 'My head is pounding')
— pressing
— prickling (as in conjunctivitis)
— scalding (cystitis)
— severe pain (gip – 'It gives me the gip')
— sharp
— shooting (sciatica, toothache)
— sickening
— smarting (burns)
— sore
— spiky
— splinter-like
— stabbing (indigestion)
— stinging (cuts, stings)
— stitch (sudden sharp pain usually due to spasm of the diaphragm)
— straining
— tearing
— tender
— throbbing (headache, an infected area)
— tingling (return of circulation to extremities)
— twinge (sudden, sharp)
— twisting.

Pain may also be described as being: acute, agonising, chronic, constant, constricting, convulsive, darting, deep-seated, difficult to move, diffuse, excruciating, fleeting, intense, intermittent, localised, mild, obstinate, persistent, radiating, severe, spasmodic, spreading, stubborn, superficial, very severe, violent.

Case history – Miss Carter

Miss Carter has had migraine attacks for many years, but recently they are coming more often and her usual tablets are not as effective. This has led to her having several days off sick from work.

Miss C.: My heads [in this context meaning the 'migraine attacks'] are getting worse. I wish I knew what brings it on [causes it].

Nurse: **When did you start having migraine?**

Miss C.: Oh, years ago when I was still at school, but now they're coming every couple of weeks.

Nurse: **How does that differ from before?**

Miss C.: I only had them once in a blue moon [very infrequently], but always when I was planning to do something special.

Nurse: **Can you think of any reasons why they're coming more often?**

Miss C.: Well, I've got a new job and it's more stressful.

Nurse: **Can you do anything about that?**

Miss C.: No chance at the moment.

Nurse: **What about things like certain foods, or drinks [in this context alcoholic drinks]. Have you noticed any link?**

Miss C.: I know to lay off [give up] chocolate. But now it's really spooky [weird, strange]. Sometimes I have a sip of wine and my head feels tight and I just know that a migraine is on its way [going to occur], and other times I have two or three glasses and get away with it [escape having a migraine attack].

Nurse: **Is it a particular type of wine?**

Miss C.: No, sometimes red and sometimes white wine.

Nurse: **Does anything special make it worse once you've got the pain?**

Miss C.: Yes, any bright light. You know like sunlight on water. It's no problem 'cos [because] I always have my dark glasses with me until I can get into bed.

Nurse: **What about the migraine attacks? Have they changed?**

Miss C.: The throbbing is much worse. It's so bad I have to lie on the bed and try to sleep.

Nurse: Do you take anything for the pain?

Miss C.: I always used to take a painkiller [analgesic] and the pain would soon go off [stop], but no joy [failure] now. Nothing seems to shift the pain [relieve the pain].

Nurse: Which painkillers?

Miss C.: Mostly Panadol [a proprietary name for paracetamol], but sometimes ibuprofen. It depends on what I have with me.

Nurse: Over the last few years much better drugs have become available for migraine.

Miss C.: Yes, I knew that, but it didn't matter while the Panadol still worked OK.

THINKING ABOUT (REFLECTION) PRACTICE: EXERCISE

Think about a recent time at work when you needed to get information, or help patients/clients/relatives to understand something to do with their care.

— Who was the person?
— What did you need to find out or tell them?
— How did you start the conversation?
— Did you get the information you needed, or were you successful in helping the person understand something?
— Did you have any difficulty understanding everything the patient/client/relative said to you?
— Do you think that they understood everything you said?
— Which parts of the communication were good and what helped to make it so?
— Which parts were less successful and what stopped them working so well?

Consider the answers you have given and pick out what you have learned from this situation. What, if anything, would you do differently if the same sort of situation happened again?

FURTHER READING

Holland K, Jenkins J, Solomon J, Whittam S 2003 Applying the Roper–Logan–Tierney model in practice. Churchill Livingstone, Edinburgh.

Roper N, Logan WW, Tierney AJ 1996 The elements of nursing, 4th edn. Churchill Livingstone, Edinburgh.

Colloquial English

6

LANGUAGE USED BY PEOPLE TO DISCUSS PROBLEMS OR SIGNS AND SYMPTOMS

Many people, especially older people, find extreme difficulty in discussing their bodily functions and signs and symptoms of a disorder with a health worker. This may be from not knowing the correct words, or shyness. Obviously, the more intimate the part of the body, the greater the embarrassment, and so a wide vocabulary of euphemisms and slang expressions has sprung up in the English language.

Quite often the person is so inarticulate that you will have to suggest various problems or symptoms and the person merely says 'yes' or 'no'. In some situations, the nurse or doctor may have to use colloquial expressions. However, there is considerable risk of misunderstanding and it is safer to use the correct terms and check that the person has understood.

Colloquial expressions show considerable regional differences. A few are included in this chapter, but it is important that you become familiar with those used locally. The expressions that people use are also influenced by their age and culture, and again you should note the expressions used locally. Those phrases which are most commonly used have been printed in italics (e.g. *back passage*). Many colloquial expressions you will hear are considered to be vulgar, offensive or discriminatory in some way. You should not use them, and those that are not commonly used in polite society, have been marked with an asterisk (*).

PARTS OF THE BODY

Anus – arse*, arsehole*, *back passage*, butt*, butthole*, hole*.
    To break wind: to fart*, to poop*, to trump*.

Bladder – waterworks, e.g. Nurse to patient: 'How are the waterworks?' or

How is your bladder working?

Bowels – gut, e.g. a pain in one's gut, to have belly ache (often used to mean bowels), to have gut ache.

Brain – head-piece, noodle, nut (e.g. use your nut).

Breast – boobs*, *bosom*, buffers*, charleys*, *chest*, chestnut*, globe*, knockers*, nipples, paps*, tits*, titties*, top part. Imitation breasts: falsies. Small breasts: 'I haven't got much'.

Buttocks – arse*, backside, *behind*, *bottom*, botty (childish), bum*, buns* (male), cheeks, hind quarters, posterior, rear, rump*, *seat*, sit-upon, stern, tail, toby.

To have large buttocks: to be broad in the beam.

Cervix – neck of womb.

Chest – to have a *flat*, barrel, *hollow*, pigeon chest.

The following are only used for females:

bosom, *breast*, buffers*, bust.

To have a bad cough: to *bark*.

Coughing: to be chesty, a bit chesty.

To have one's chest finger-tapped: to have a thump.

Clitoris – clit*.

Crotch – often used to mean groin or skin covering genitalia.

Ear – bat ears (prominent), a cauliflower ear (from boxing), flappers, lug* (e.g. to have lugache*).

Rather deaf: to be hard of hearing.

Elbow – *funny bone*, e.g. *to hit one's funny bone* (so called because of the strange tingling one experiences when it is struck).

Enlargement of abdomen in older people – middle-age spread.

Eyes – glimmers*, ogles*, optics, peepers.

To have a squint: to be boss-eyed, to be cock-eyed, to be wall-eyed.

To have low visual acuity in one eye: to have a lazy eye.

Face – clock*, dial*, mug*, physog*.

Genitals – male and female: bits, package, *down below*, *private* *parts*, thing, pencil and tassle* (male child's penis and scrotum).

Hand – mitt, paw.

Head – bonce; brain-box, brain-pan, napper, nob, noddle, nous-box (nous means intelligence, common sense), nut, *skull*.

Heart – engine, e.g. 'my engine's not working properly', jam tart* (Cockney), ticker.

Something wrong with one's heart: *to have a dicky heart*.

To have a weak heart: to have a heart.

Hymen – cherry, maidenhead, maid's ring (Cockney).

Intestines – bowels, guts, innards, *inside*.

Legs – bandy legged (bow), drumsticks (very thin), K-legged (with knees knocking together), knock-kneed (knees bent inwards to face each other), peg leg (an artificial leg), pins, spindles.

A lame leg: to have a gammy leg.

Short legs: to have duck's disease.

Walk badly: to be bad on one's pins.

Walking with the feet turned in: hen-toed.

Lungs – bellows, tubes.

To be bad in one's breathing: *to be short-winded*.

Mouth – chops*, gob* trap*.

Navel – belly button.

Neck – Adam's apple (projection of thyroid cartilage of larynx), salt cellars (very deep hollows above collar-bone in female neck), scruff of neck (nape).

Nose – beacon* (red and large), beak*, conk*, hooter*, sniffer*, snitch*.

Nasal congestion: to be blocked up, bunged up, *stuffy*.

Nasal discharge: snot*.

Noisy breathing in children due to nasal congestion: snuffles.

Running nose: a snotty nose*.

Penis – almond*, almond rock* (Cockney), bean*, button* (baby), club*, cock*, dick*, equipment*, gear*, it*, John Thomas*, knob*, little man*, little tail* (small boys), meat*, old man*, Peter*, pinkle*, prick*, *private parts*, *privates*, rod*, shaft*, she*, stick*, tadger* (Northern England), tassel*, thing*, tool*, Will*, Willie*.

Scrotum – bag*, sac.

Skull – brain pan.

Spine – backbone.

Stomach – abdomen, belly, bread-basket*, corporation (when large), croop, guts (stomach and intestines), innards, inner man, peenie, pinafore, *tummy*.

To belch: *to burp*.

The noise the stomach makes when one is hungry: *to have stomach rumbles*.

Something wrong with it: to have a gastric stomach.

Stomach ache: to have a pain in one's guts.

Teeth – buck teeth (protruding); peggy, peggies (childish).

Testes/testicles – ballocks*, balls*, bollocks*, charleys*, cobblers*, cods*, nuts*, pills*, pillocks*, stones*. See **Genitals.**

Throat – clack*, gullet, organ-pipe (windpipe).

A very severe cough: a churchyard cough.

Sputum: *phlegm*.

To be hoarse: *to have a frog in the throat*.

To have a sore throat: to have a throat.

Tongue – clack*, clapper*.

The tongue can be described as: coated, dirty, *furred*, furry, thick.

Talkative person: *a chatterbox*.

Trachea – *windpipe*.

Umbilicus – belly button (childish), *navel*.

Urethra – pipe, waterpipe.

Uterus – box, *womb*.

Vagina (or vulva) – birth canal, box*, brush*, crack*, cunt*, *down below*, fanny*, *front passage*, hair pie*, it, private (e.g. 'my private is sore'), *private part*, pussy*, slit*, thing*, there, twat*, up inside.

BODY FUNCTIONS

Constipation, to have – to be bunged up, to be costive, *I haven't been for 4 days*. I haven't had a road through me for a week*.

Defaecate, to – to crap*, to do a big job, to do a job, to do a pooh (childish), to do a rear*, to do number two, to do one's business, to go to the toilet (and use paper), to have a clear out, *to have the bowels opened*, to job*, *to pass one's motions*, to shit*, *to use a bedpan* (hospital).

Diarrhoea, to have – the trots, collywobbles, Gippy tummy, run'ems, runs, scours, squitters.

To have a sudden attack of diarrhoea: *to be taken short*.

Die, to – to be a goner, to be all over, to be slipping (to be dying), to burn oneself out (die early through overwork), to conk out, to go (go away), to go home, to go to the next world, to hang up one's hat, to have had it, to have one's number up, to have had one's chips, to have one foot in the grave (to be dying), to kick the bucket, *to pass away*, to peg out, to pip out, to pop off (usually die suddenly), to push up daisies, to snuff it or out, to turn it in, to turn one's toes up, *to have had a long (or good) innings* (to die at an old age), *to lay out* (prepare for burial or cremation).

Note: To commit suicide: to kill oneself.

Faint, to – *to black out*, *to have a black-out*, to go off hooks, to pass out.

Faeces, stools – baby's yellow (infantile excrement), business, cack*, job*, mess*, *motions*, number two, shit*.

Nurse to patient: 'Are your motions well formed?'.

Mothers often say of a child: 'His toilet is green' (meaning his stools are green).

Note that 'a dose of salts' means Epsom salts.

Tenesmus: *straining*.

Impotent, to become – to be no good to one's wife, to lose one's nature.

A man's impotence will be expressed by his wife/partner in the following ways: he can't sustain an erection, *he can't manage*, his cock's soft or droopy*. Doctor to man: 'Can you get a hard on?'.

Menstruate, to – to be unwell, *one's period*, the curse, the days, the monthlies, the other, the thing, *the time of the month*, the usual.

'Have you seen anything?' (feminine euphemism).

'I haven't seen for 6 weeks' (no menstruation, possibly pregnant).

Nurse to patient: 'When was your last period?'

Naked, to be – to be in one's birthday suit, to be in the altogether, to be starkers.

Pregnant, to be – away the trip* (Scottish working class), to be caught*, *to be expecting*, *to be having a baby*, to be in a delicate condition, to be in an interesting condition, to be in Kittle (Scottish), to be in pig*, to be in pod*, to be in the club*, to be in the family way, to be in the pudding club*, to be one in line*, to be preggers*, to be up the duff*, to be up the pole*, to be up the stick*, to catch on, to catch the virus*, to click*, to cop it*, to fall for a baby (to have an unwanted pregnancy), to have a bun in the oven*, to have a touch of the sun*.

She's 6 months pregnant: she's 6 months gone.

Sleep, to – to close one's eyes, *to doze* (short sleep), to go off (to fall asleep), to go to the land of nod, *to have a catnap* (short sleep), *to have a doze*, *to have a snooze* (short sleep), *to have forty winks* (short sleep), *to have some shut-eye*, *to nod off* (short sleep), ziz.

Urinate, to (micturate) – to do number one, *to go to the loo*, to have a run-out, *to pass water*, to pee, to pee-wee (childish), to piddle*, to piss*, *to spend a penny* (women only), to tiddle (childish), to tinkle (women only), to wee-wee (childish).

Nocturia: to get up in the night to pass urine.

Hostess to guests: 'Do you want to wash your hands?' (Do you want to go to the toilet?).

The lavatory can be described as: *bathroom*, bog*, *cloakroom*, convenience, *Gents'*, heads*, *Ladies'*, lav, lavvy, little girls' room, *loo*, place, powder room (Ladies' in a hotel), privies, rears*, *toilet*, WC.

A chamber pot: banjo*, gerry*, po, pot, potty (childish).

To hold a baby over a chamber pot: to hold out a baby.

To put a baby on a chamber pot: to pot.

Vomit, to – to be ill, *to be sick*, to bring up, to lose the lot, to puke*, to pump your heart up, to sick up, to spew*, to throw up*.

Nausea: the sicks.

To have nausea: to feel queasy, *to feel sick*.

'Have you vomited?' '*Have you been sick?*'

To try to vomit but nothing comes up: *to retch*.

To vomit very much: to be as sick as a dog (or cat).

To have a headache and vomiting: to have a sick headache.

Weep, to – to blub, to blubber, to break down, *to cry*, to turn on the waterworks, to turn the tap on.

MENTAL AND PHYSICAL STATES

Angry, to be – to be cross, to be crusty, to be heated, to be hot under the collar, to be liverish, to be livid, to be shirty, to be steamed up, to flip, to fly off the handle, to go off the deep end, to have a paddy, to have a tantrum, to jump down someone's throat, to let off steam, to lose one's hair, to lose one's shirt, to play the devil, to see red.

Confused, to be – to be all at sea, befuddled, bewildered, disorientated, flummoxed, forgetful, muddled, muzzy, unsure.

Depressed, to be – to be blue, to be browned-off, to be down in the dumps, to be down in the hips, to be down in the mouth, to be fed up, to be low, to be off the hinges, to have a button on, to have a chopper, to have a face as long as a fiddle, to have the droops, to have the hump, to have the hyp, to have the mopes, to have the pip.

Drunk, to be – to be a dipso (dipsomaniac), to be boozed (boozy), to be fou*, to be fresh (slightly drunk), to be fuddled (confused with drink), to be high on surge (to be drunk on surgical spirit), to be lush (slightly drunk), to be merry (happy with drink), to be muzzed, to be on the bottle (habitual drinker), to be paralytic (very drunk), to be pie-eyed, to be plastered, to be slewed, to be sloshed, to be soaked (very drunk), to be sozzled (very drunk), to be squiffy (slightly drunk), to be tiddly (slightly drunk), to be tight, to be tipsy (slightly drunk), to be under the influence (of liquor), to be well-oiled, to be woozy (confused with drink), to have a skinful (very drunk), to have Dutch courage (extra courage induced by alcohol), to have more than one can carry, to have one over the eight, to see pink elephants (or spiders) (to suffer from DTs), to have a hangover (to feel ill as a result of alcohol), to have a morning-after-the-night-before (to feel ill as a result of alcohol), to hit the bottle (to drink excessively).

Dull, to be – to be a dream, a drip, a moron, a muggins, a noodle, a pie-can, a sap*, a wet, dead alive, dopey, dumb, foolish, goofy, half-baked, half-witted, lethargic, mutton-headed, silly, simple, slack, slow, soft, stupid, thick, thick-skulled.

Exhausted, to be – to be all in, to be clapped out*, to be dead, to be done for, done in, done up, to be fagged out, to be finished, to be flaked out, to be jiggered, to be knackered*, to be knocked up, to be ready to drop, to be shagged*, to be shattered, *to be tired out*, to be used up (utterly exhausted), *to be weary*, to be whacked, to feel like death, to go all to pieces (collapse from exhaustion).

To knock it out of one, 'walking uphill knocks it out of me' (walking uphill exhausts me).

Healthy, to be – to be A1, to be as fit as a box of birds, to be as fit as a fiddle, to be fighting fit, to be first rate, to be full of beans, to be in fine fettle, to be in the pink, to be on good form, to have plenty of pep (pep = energy), to have plenty of vim (energy, vigour), to perk up (recover good health).

To begin to recover after an illness: *to be on the mend*, to turn the corner.

Madness – (in varying degrees): to be a bit touched, to be a case, to be a character (to be eccentric, odd), a scatterbrain (very forgetful, vague), to be as mad as a hatter, balmy, (barmy), bats, batty, bonkers, to be clean gone, cracked, crackers, crack-pot, crank, crazy, to be dippy, dotty, gaga (senile), goofy, half-baked, kinky, loony, loopy, mad, to be mental, non compos mentis, not all there, to be not right in one's head, nuts, off one's block, off one's chump, off one's head, off one's nut, off one's rocker, to be off the rails, out of one's mind, to be peculiar, potty, round the bend, scatty, a screwball, screwy, silly, simple, soft, stupid, up the creek, weak in the upper storey, to go doolally, to go hay-wire, to have bats in the belfry, with a tile (or screw) missing (or loose).

Psychiatric (mental) hospital: bin, funny farm, loony bin, nuthouse.

Nervous, to feel – to be a fuss-pot, to be a jitter-bug, to be all hot and bothered, to be all of a dither, to be chewed up, *to be edgy*, on edge, to be fidgety, to be in a blue funk, to be in a flap, to be in a stew, to be in a tizzy, to be jittery, to be screwed up, to be shook-up (nerve-racked), to get all het-up, *to get in a state*, to get uptight, to go all hot and cold, to go into a flat spin, to go to pieces (collapse through nerves), to go up the wall, to have ants in one's pants*, to have butterflies in one's stomach, to have forty fits, to have kittens, to have the creeps, to have the heebie-jeebies, to have the shakes, to have the shivers, to have the twitters, to have the willies, to have the wind up, to have the worrits, to lose one's cool, to worrit (be anxious).

Unwell, to be – to be anyhow, to be below par, to be groggy, to be not oneself, to be not quite right, *to be off colour*, to be out of sorts, to be peaky, to be pingley, to be poorly, *to be run down*, to be taken bad, to be tenpence to the bob, *to be under the weather*, to be washed-out, to be weedy (anaemic, sickly), to be wobbly (weak after an illness), to be wonky (weak), to come all over queer, faint, ill (suddenly feel unwell), to crack up, to feel a bit off it, to feel a bit rough, to feel funny, to feel half-baked, to feel like death warmed up (very unwell), to feel like nothing on earth, to feel lousy, to feel queer, to feel ragged, to feel seedy, to go funny, to have a bad turn.

Vertigo – *to be dizzy*, to be giddy, to be muzzy, to feel the room spin, to feel queer, to have a mazy bout, to have a swimming head.

GENERAL EXPRESSIONS

(In this section the text in bold type is the colloquial expression.)

Dope, physic – any kind of medicine.

Medicine – anything taken to relieve pain or symptoms of illness. Usually the word refers to liquid or drugs taken by mouth.

Pills, tablets – drugs in tablet form. *Note:* to be on the pill: to be taking the contraceptive pill.

A tonic – medicine to invigorate one after an illness.

To be at death's door, to be critical, to be nearly a goner – to be dangerously ill.

To be laid up – to be confined to bed, e.g. 'I was laid up for 3 months'.

To be looking up – to improve.

To be off sick, to be on the sick-list, having a sicky – to be absent from work due to illness.

To be on the mend – to improve.

To be nesh, to be soft – to be prone to illness.

To be under a doctor – to be in a doctor's care.

To find one's legs – to begin to walk after an illness.

To get a chit from the doctor – to get a medical certificate.

To go under – to have a general anaesthetic.

To have a bad turn – to become ill suddenly.

To have a bug, a germ – to have an infection.

To have a check-up – to be medically examined, or have a screening test.

To have a jab – to have an injection.

To have a set-back – to have a relapse.

To have a temperature – to be pyrexial or feverish, to have a high temperature, e.g. 'I've had a temperature all day'.

To have gas – to have a general anaesthetic.

To have painkillers – to have analgesics.

To have sleeping pills – to have sedatives.

To have time off – to have sick leave.

To stitch – to suture.

To suck lozenges – to suck small tablets, usually for coughs and sore throat.

To take a turn for the better – to improve.

To take medicine for the bowels – to take a laxative.

To take stitches out – to remove sutures.

To turn the corner – to improve.

REPRODUCTIVE AND SEXUAL HEALTH PROBLEMS

The vocabulary to express menstruation and pregnancy is listed separately under body functions (see p. 126–129).

Women's health expressions

Abortion (*Note:* In practice it is usual to refer to an abortion as a 'miscarriage' to avoid causing distress, as some women will associate the term abortion with a deliberate termination of pregnancy) – spontaneous miscarriage, a miscarriage, a miss*. 'It came away.' 'I lost my baby' or 'We lost our baby.'

Candidiasis – vaginal thrush.

Confinement – childbirth, delivery. 'Did you have an easy confinement?'

Dilatation and curettage – *D&C*, a scrape, e.g. 'I've had two D&Cs' (two scrapes).

Dysmenorrhoea – period pains, to be unwell.

Efforts to terminate a pregnancy – to bring on a period, to lose it (a baby), to get rid of a baby. 'They took the baby away.'

Episiotomy – to make a perineal cut. 'I'm going to cut you now.'

Flooding – excessive bleeding from the uterus during menstruation.

Hot flushes and night sweats, to have – to have a feeling of being hot, looking hot and red, and sometimes sweaty. Associated with the menopause.

Hysterectomy – to have an internal operation, to have a major operation, to have all taken away (uterus and ovaries).

Menarche – the beginning of menstrual periods, e.g. 'When did your periods start?'.

Menopause – the end of periods, e.g. 'When did your periods end?', the change, that certain age, the time of life.
I haven't seen anything for 6 months.
It's your age. It's the time of life.

Menorrhagia – heavy periods.

Parturition – labour, to be in labour. 'How often are you having contractions?'

Placenta – the afterbirth.

Repair of the prolapse – 'I was stitched up below', to be hitched up.

Rupture the membranes, to – to break my waters.

Sanitary towels – pads, STs, Tampax (a brand of tampons worn internally), towels, wings.

Still-born baby – baby born dead.

Suture – to be stitched up.

Termination of pregnancy – an abortion. 'I don't want this baby. Can I have an abortion?' 'I did away with it.'* 'I decided not to go ahead with the pregnancy.'

Vaginal discharge – to have whites, to lose down there. 'Something comes away from me ...'

Version – turning (of fetus).

Men's health expressions

Coitus interruptus – *to be careful*, to withdraw. 'My husband's very careful.'

Ejaculate, to – to come, to get your rocks off*, to shoot.

Erection, to have an – to have a hard on, to have a stand*, to have a stiff*, to have the horn*.

Impotent (now known as erectile dysfunction), to be – to have a half-stand*. 'I can't keep it up.' 'My husband has trouble.'

Impotent, to become – to lose one's nature.

Semen – come, cum, jizz.

Sexual health expressions

Anal intercourse – buggery, bumming*. 'He wants to come at me from behind.'* To rim*.

Bisexual – AC–DC*, to be double-jointed*.

Dyspareunia – *love pain.*

Female homosexual/lesbian – to be gay, kinky*, to be butch (a lesbian with male characteristics), a dyke*, a lessie*.

French kiss – kiss with mouth open and insert tongue in partner's mouth.

Heterosexual – straight.

Homosexual expressions – to be the active/passive partner, eating ass*, reaming*, tonguing (using the mouth on anus), finger fucking*, fisting* (using finger/fist in anal canal).

Illegitimate, to be – to be a bastard, to be born on the wrong side of the blanket, to get into trouble (unmarried pregnancy), to have a natural child.

Male homosexual – bent*, a fag*, a faggot*, a fairy*, a nancy-boy*, a pansy*, a pouf*, a poufter*, a queen*, *a queer*, *gay*, kinky*.

Oral sex – blow job*, give head*, to go down on someone, rimming*, sixty-nine* (mutual oral sex), to suck off.

Orgasm – climax.
   To experience an orgasm: *to come*, to have a thrill. 'When I come.' 'When he's finished.'

Sexual intercourse – intimacy, to do it, to fuck*, to get it with, to get layed, to go with someone, *to go to bed with someone*, to have it, *to have sex*, to knock up*, *to make love*, to perform, to shag*, to roger, to screw*, *to sleep with*.

To have a regular sexual partner – to go steady. 'We're an item.'

To masturbate – to beat off*, to bring oneself off*, to fiddle*, to jack off*, to jerk off*, to rub up*, to shag*, to shake*, to toss*, to wank* (wanker: masturbator).

To neck – hug and kiss intimately.

To pet – kiss and caress extensively.

Sexual intercourse is often referred to as *a normal married life* by older people. Note the negative use, such as 'We can't have a normal married life'. Also, 'He doesn't trouble me', meaning the husband/partner does not demand sexual intercourse if the woman does not want it. 'He doesn't bother about that sort of thing' implies a not very demanding partner. 'He wants it too often' means a demanding one.

Phrases such as, '*When I go with my husband*', *When we have it*', '*When we have sex*', 'When he does it' are most commonly used.

Family planning, contraception

Condom – briefs (short condoms), Durex (trade name often used as a synonym), envelope, French letter, Johnny*, jolly bag*, rubber*, sheath, skin.

Diaphragm – Dutch cap, cap.

Emergency contraception – morning after pill.

Female condom.

Intrauterine contraceptive devices (IUCDs) – the coil.

Oral contraceptive – the pill.

Assisted conception, fertility clinic

Frequency of sexual intercourse – 'How often do you try for a baby?', 'When and how often do you have intercourse?'

In vitro fertilisation (IVF) – test tube baby.

Tubal insufflation – I had my tubes blown.

Sexually transmitted (acquired) infections (STIs, SAIs)

Gonorrhoea – clap, gleet, morning drop, strain, tear, a dose, the whites, to catch a cold.

Primary syphilis – bumps (African Caribbean).

Pubic lice – crabs, to be chatty*.

Seminal fluid – your husband's fluid.

Sexual health centre/clinic – GUM clinic, special clinic, VD clinic

Syphilis – bad blood, lues, pox, siff.

Expressions:

To have a double event (syphilis and gonorrhoea).

To piss pins and needles*.

Scalded (infected with gonorrhoea).

Expressions used by patients:

I've been to the GUM clinic.

I've picked up something.

I'm afraid I've got it.

I've caught (or got) something.

I've got a dose (gonorrhoea).

I've got a full house* (syphilis and gonorrhoea).

I've got genital warts.

I've got trouble down below.

I've noticed something odd.

I've got trouble with my meat*.

I've been after the girls (or men).

Note: 'The whites' may be used by women to mean any white vaginal discharge.

African Caribbean individuals may use 'scratch' for irritate or itch, e.g. 'It scratches me' means 'It irritates and I want to scratch'.

Prostitutes (sex workers) may say, 'I'm a business/working girl', 'I'm on the game'.

The health professional in the sexual health clinic will ask: 'Have you any discharge?', 'Does it irritate?', 'Do you have pain when you pass water?', 'Have you any swelling?', 'Have you a sore place?', 'Have you a rash?'.

GLOSSARY OF MEDICAL AND COLLOQUIAL NAMES

Medical name	*Colloquial name*
Alopecia	baldness
Arteriosclerosis	hardening of the arteries
Blepharitis	sore eyelids

Bursitis	housemaid's knee, tennis elbow (see epicondylitis)
Cancer	a growth, the big C, the worst, tumour
Candidiasis; monilia	thrush
Cerebral palsy	to be spastic
Cerebrovascular accident	stroke
Colic	gripes
Concussion	KO'd, to be concussed, to be knocked out
Conjunctivitis	pink eye
Contusion	bruise
Convulsions	fits
Coronary thrombosis; myocardial infarction	a coronary, heart attack
Coryza	cold
Dandruff	scurf
Delirium tremens	DTs, the jerks, the shakes
Diabetes mellitus	sugar diabetes
Dysmenorrhoea	painful periods
Dysphagia	difficulty swallowing
Dyspnoea	breathless, out of breath, panting, puffed, short of breath
Dyspepsia	indigestion
Encephalitis	brain fever
Enuresis	bed-wetting
Epicondylitis	golfer's elbow (medial side), tennis elbow (lateral side)
Epistaxis	nosebleeds
Eructation	belching
Erythema pernio	chilblains
Flatulence, flatus	wind. *Note:* To belch (to send out wind from stomach noisily), to fart* (to send out wind from anus)

Frequency	I keep wanting to go (to pass urine)
Furuncle	boil
Gonorrhoea	clap
Haemorrhoids	piles
Halitosis	bad breath
Hernia	rupture
Herpes simplex	cold blister or sore
Herpes zoster	shingles
Hordeolum	stye
Hydrophobia	rabies
Hypertension	high blood pressure
Incontinence	leaky, not to be able to hold one's water or motions, to have an accident
Infectious mononucleosis	glandular fever
Influenza	flu
Leucorrhoea	whites
Menopause	the change (of life), the turn (of life)
Menstruation	period(s)
Myopia	short-sight
Neuralgia	face ache
Nocturia	to get up at night (to pass water)
Oedema	dropsy, swelling
Osteoporosis	brittle bone disease
Parotitis (infectious)	mumps
Pediculosis capitis; head lice	nits
Peritonsillar abscess	quinsy
Pertussis	whooping cough
Poliomyelitis	infantile paralysis, polio
Pruritus	itching
Pyrexia	fever, a high temperature
Pyrosis	heartburn, water-brash

Rheumatic disease	screws, springes, rheumatics
Rubella	German measles
Rubeola; morbilli	measles
Scarlatina	scarlet fever
Seizure	convulsion, fit
Strabismus	a squint
Syncope	fainting
Tachycardia	palpitations
Tendonitis	golfer's elbow, tennis elbow
Tetanus	lockjaw
Tinea circinata	ringworm
Tinnitus	ringing in the ears
Tuberculosis	TB
Urticaria	heat spots, hives, nettle rash
Varicella	chickenpox
Verrucae	warts
Vesicle	blister

Idioms: parts of the body

7

INTRODUCTION

The English language has thousands of idioms. By an 'idiom' we mean a number of words which, when taken together, have a different meaning from that of each separate word.

The reason for including these idioms of parts of the body is that, although you may never need to use them yourself, you should be able to recognise them. You may be told by a person that by the end of the day he is 'on his knees' and you must realise that he is using the word 'knee' idiomatically. What he means is that he is extremely tired after work and feels like collapsing.

A woman may tell you of her worries and say she has just managed to 'keep her head above water'. If you are not familiar with the idiom, you may think she has tried to save herself from drowning but, in fact, she means that she is terribly short of money and is having a struggle to keep out of debt.

Words and phrases connected with parts of the body have also been included, such as 'chesty', 'throaty' and 'to speak through one's nose'. It is essential that you understand these.

IDIOMS: PARTS OF THE BODY

Figures 7.1 to 7.3 are provided so you can familiarise yourself with the words usually used in everyday conversation to describe parts of the body.

Arm

A shot in the arm: something that does a person good.

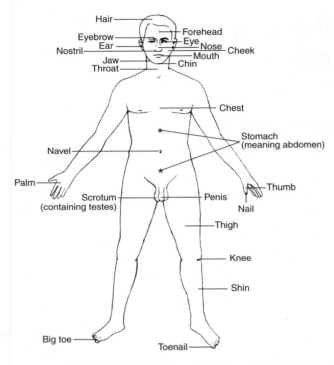

Fig. 7.1 Parts of the body (male front view). Reproduced with permission from Parkinson, *Manual of English for the Overseas Doctor*, 5th edn. Churchill Livingstone, 1999.

To give one's right arm (usually with *would*): to be willing to make a sacrifice to get something.

To keep someone at arm's length: to avoid being friendly.

To stand by with folded arms: to do nothing when action seems necessary.

To welcome someone with open arms: to greet warmly.

Back

To back a horse: to place money on a horse in a race, to bet.

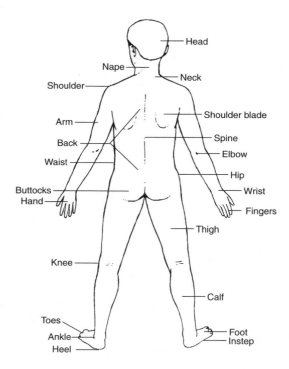

Fig. 7.2 Parts of the body (back view). Reproduced with permission from Parkinson, *Manual of English for the Overseas Doctor*, 5th edn. Churchill Livingstone, 1999.

To back down: to be less demanding than before; to withdraw one's claim.

To back out: to withdraw from.

To back someone or something: to give one's support.

To be on one's back: to be ill in bed.

To break one's back: to overwork.

To do something behind someone's back: to act deceitfully.

To have one's back to the wall: to be struggling against great difficulties.

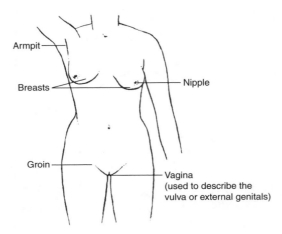

Fig. 7.3 Parts of the body (female front view). Reproduced with permission from Parkinson, *Manual of English for the Overseas Doctor*, 5th edn. Churchill Livingstone, 1999.

To put (get, set) someone's back up: to make someone angry.

To see the back of someone/something: to get rid of someone/ something that is annoying, unpleasant.

To turn one's back on: to abandon, to refuse to help.

Blood

A young blood: dashing young man.

Bad blood: ill feeling (between people, nations).

Blood is thicker than water: one's own relations come before all other people.

His blood is up: he is in a fighting mood.

His blood ran cold in his veins: he was filled with terror.

It is more than flesh and blood can stand: too much for human beings to endure.

One's own flesh and blood: one's own family.

To do something in cold blood: deliberately; when one is not angry.

To get blood out of a stone: to get pity from someone hard; to achieve the impossible.

To get someone's blood up: to provoke someone very much.

To have fresh, new blood: to have new members in a business, family or society.

To make one's blood boil: to make one very angry.

To run in the blood: to have an inherited quality.

Bone

A bone of contention: the subject of constant disagreement.

He will never make old bones: will not live to an old age.

To be all skin and bones: very thin.

To be bone dry: completely dry.

To be bone-idle: completely idle, lazy.

To bone up on: to study intensively.

To feel something in one's bones: to feel quite sure about something intuitively.

To have a bone to pick with someone: to wish to complain about something.

To make no bones about doing something: to have no hesitation in doing something (usually unpleasant).

To work one's fingers to the bone: to work very hard without appreciation.

Brain

A brain-child: original idea of a person or group.

A brain drain: movement of trained and qualified workers to other countries (usually for better conditions).

A brainstorm: cerebral disturbance; a mental aberration.

A brainstorming session: a method of solving problems in which many people suggest ideas which are then discussed.

A brain-teaser: problem, puzzle.

A brainwave: a sudden inspiration or clever idea.

A scatter-brained person: a careless, forgetful person.

Brain-fag: mental exhaustion.

Brain fever: encephalitis.

Brainwashing: forcing someone to change his beliefs by use of extreme mental pressure.

Brainless: foolish, stupid.

Brainy: clever.

To *blow one's brain out:* to shoot oneself in the head.

To *have something on the brain:* to be obsessive about something.

To *pick someone's brains:* to find out someone's good ideas and use them.

To *rack one's brains:* to think very hard; to solve a problem or remember something.

Breast

To *make a clean breast of something:* to confess everything.

Brow (forehead), Brows (arch of hair above eyes)

A *high-brow:* someone interested in intellectual matters and culture.

A *low-brow:* someone showing little interest in intellectual matters and culture.

To *browbeat someone into doing something:* to intimidate someone with severe looks and words, to bully.

To *knit one's brows:* to frown.

Cheek

Cheek: disrespectful speech, impudence.

Cheeks: buttocks.

To *be cheeky:* to be disrespectful, impudent.

To *cheek someone:* to speak impudently to someone.

To *have the cheek to do something:* to be bold, rude enough to do something.

To *turn the other cheek:* to refuse to retaliate.

Chest

To be chesty: to have trouble with one's lungs.

To cock one's chest: to boast about oneself.

To get something off one's chest: to free one's mind by speaking about something that was troubling one.

Get that across your chest!: Eat that! (usually a large, nourishing meal). Slang.

To puff one's chest out: to be proud of oneself.

Chin

A chin: a talk.

Chin up: be brave.

To be up to the chin in work, etc.: to have too much work to do.

To chin: to talk, to gossip.

To have a chin-wag: to talk with friends about unimportant matters, to chatter.

To keep one's chin up: to be brave, to be cheerful in the face of difficulties.

To take something on the chin: to suffer severe difficulties with courage.

Ears

In at one ear and out at the other: ignored or quickly forgotten advice.

To be all ears: to listen very carefully.

To be up to one's ears in: deeply involved or occupied in.

To box someone's ears: to smack someone on the ears.

To come to one's ears: to hear a rumour.

To earmark: to put someone/something aside for a special purpose.

To fall on deaf ears: to pass unnoticed.

To give one's ears for something: to be prepared to do anything to get what one desires.

To have a person's ear: to have the favourable attention of someone.

To have a word in someone's ear: to speak in private.

To keep one's ear to the ground: to listen carefully.

To play it by ear: to do what seems best at the time.

To prick up one's ears: to have one's attention suddenly aroused.

To send someone away with a flea in his ear: to criticise someone severely so that he goes away unhappily.

To set people by the ears: to cause them to quarrel.

To turn a deaf ear: to ignore, pretend not to hear.

Elbow

Elbow-grease: vigorous polishing; hard physical work.

Elbow-room: plenty of room to move freely.

Out-at-elbows: of a coat, worn out; of a person, poor.

To elbow one's way through a crowd: to push with one's elbows.

To raise the elbow: to drink too much.

Eye

A blue-eyed boy: a pet, a favourite.

A sight for sore eyes: someone or something very welcome, pleasant.

An eye for an eye: to punish those who hurt us.

An eye-opener: an event or piece of news which causes surprise.

An eyesore: a very unpleasant thing to look at.

Eyeball to eyeball: face to face with someone.

Eye contact: looking directly into another person's eyes.

Eye-opener: an enlightening experience.

Eye-wash: lotion for bathing eyes; words or actions intended to mislead.

Green-eyed: jealous.

In the eyes of: in the opinion of.

In the mind's eye: imagining in the mind.

In the public eye: to be watched by the public constantly.

The apple of one's eye: someone or something very precious.

To be up to the eyes in work: to have far too much work to do.

To catch someone's eye: to attract someone's attention.

To cry one's eyes out: to weep very much.

To do something with one's eyes open: to act knowing the results of the action.

To eye someone: to look at carefully, admiringly, jealously, etc.

To get (or give) a black eye: to receive (or give) a blow on the eye so that the skin around it goes black.

To give someone the glad eye: to encourage someone to be amorous.

To have an eye for: to have a liking or ability to do something; to have good judgement on something.

To have an eye on/to the main chance: to think and work with one's own advantage always in view.

To have half an eye on: not to give something one's full attention.

To have one's eyes opened: to be forced to see reality.

To keep an eye on someone/something: to watch carefully.

To keep one's eye open for: to watch carefully.

To keep one's eyes skinned: to be very watchful.

To make eyes at someone: to look at someone (usually of the opposite sex) with open admiration and invitation.

To pull the wool over someone's eyes: to try to hide the truth from someone.

To run one's eye over: to look quickly at, to glance at.

To see eye to eye with someone: to agree; to have the same ideas.

To turn a blind eye: to ignore deliberately, pretend not to see.

Face

Face-ache: neuralgia.

Let's face it: let's be honest with each other.

To be a slap in the face: a sudden disappointment, rejection.

To face the music: to face criticism/punishment as a result of one's own actions.

To face up to something: to meet courageously (usually difficulties).

To *fly in the face of convention, rules, etc.:* to defy, disobey openly.

To *have a face as long as a fiddle:* to look depressed.

To *keep a straight face:* not laugh. (Often used negatively, e.g. 'I couldn't keep a straight face'.)

To *look someone in the face:* to look directly at someone.

To *lose face:* to be humiliated, to be put to shame.

To *make/pull a face:* to grimace.

To *pull a long face:* to look depressed, disappointed, displeased.

To *put a brave/good face on it:* to behave as if circumstances are better than they really are.

To *put one's face on:* to apply cosmetics to one's face.

To *save one's face:* to try to avoid shaming oneself openly.

To *set one's face against:* to oppose.

To *show one's face:* to appear, be seen.

To *stare one in the face:* something that is obvious, clear to see.

Feet – see Foot

Fingers

Not to raise (lift, stir) a finger to help someone: to refuse to be of any help.

One's fingers itch to do something: one wishes very much to do something.

To *be all fingers and thumbs:* to be clumsy with one's hands often due to nervousness.

To *be light-fingered:* to steal easily.

To *burn one's fingers:* to get into trouble by interfering in other people's affairs.

To *finger:* to touch.

To *get/pull one's finger out:* to stop being lazy, work harder (slang).

To *have a finger in every pie:* to be involved in many activities.

To *have butter fingers:* to let things slip out of the hands.

To *have something at one's fingertips:* to know perfectly.

To keep one's fingers crossed (for someone): hope for luck with a problem or difficulty.

To lay/put one's finger on something: to realise the most important aspect of a matter.

To let something slip through one's fingers: to lose hold of, allow to escape (usually of opportunities).

To twist a person round one's finger: to have someone in one's power so that they do all one wishes.

Flesh

Flesh wound: one not reaching bone or a vital organ.

One's own flesh and blood: one's own family.

Proud flesh: new flesh coming from a wound.

Sins of the flesh: sexual sins.

To be neither fish nor flesh: to be of indefinite character.

To have one's pound of flesh: to insist cruelly on repayment.

To lose flesh: to get thinner.

To make one's flesh creep: to be terrified so that one's skin seems to move.

To put on flesh: to get fatter.

To see someone in the flesh: actually to see someone.

Foot, feet

My foot!: Nonsense! Rubbish!

Not to let the grass grow under one's feet: to act quickly when one has made a decision.

To be on one's feet: to be in reasonable health; to be standing.

To be run off one's feet: to be so busy one cannot sit down.

To dog one's footsteps: to follow one constantly and so cause irritation.

To drag one's feet: to be slow to take action.

To fall on one's feet: to be lucky.

To fall over one's feet to be kind, helpful, etc.: to make a great effort to be kind, helpful, etc.

To find one's feet: to be comfortably settled in a new job, situation, etc.

To foot the bill: to pay.

To get cold feet: to be afraid, discouraged.

To go on foot: to walk.

To have one foot in the grave: to be very ill, close to death.

To have one's feet on the ground: to be practical, sensible.

To have the world at one's feet: to be very successful.

To put one's best foot forward: to walk quickly, to work quickly.

To put one's feet up: to relax, to rest.

To put one's foot down: to be firm, to protest.

To put one's foot in it: to do or say something that causes anger, trouble.

To set someone on his feet: to help, usually with money, to start a business, etc.

To stand on one's own feet: to be independent.

To step off on the wrong foot: to start something in the wrong way.

Hair

A hair's breadth: a very small distance.

Hair-raising (stories): terrifying.

Not turn a hair: to show no sign of fear or emotional upset.

To a hair: exactly (usually of weight).

To get in a person's hair: to annoy, irritate someone.

To have one's hair standing on end: to be terrified.

To have someone by the short hairs: to have control over them.

To keep one's hair on: not to grow angry.

To let down one's hair: to act freely, to be uninhibited.

To split hairs: to argue about very small, unimportant differences.

Hand

A right-hand man: someone who can be relied on for help and advice.

At first hand: directly.

Hands off!: Do not touch.

Hands-on experience: involving active participation.

Never to do a hand's turn: never make the slightest effort.

To be a handful: to be difficult to control.

To be an old hand at something: to be experienced.

To be hand-in-glove with someone: to be extremely friendly (usually planning something together).

To be high-handed: to be arrogant.

To be offhand: to be abrupt in manner, casual.

To be off one's hands: to no longer be responsible for someone or something.

To be open-handed: to be generous with money.

To be out of hand (of children, a situation, etc.): to be out of control.

To be underhand: to be deceitful, dishonest, not open.

To eat out of someone's hand: to do whatever one wishes.

To force someone's hand: to make someone do something.

To get one's hand in: to get to know how to do something.

To give/lend someone a hand: to help someone physically.

To give someone a free hand: to allow someone to do as he wishes.

To hand: to give, to offer.

To have a hand in something: to share in the activity.

To have one's hands full: to be extremely busy.

To have one's hands tied: to be unable to act in the way one wishes.

To have the upper hand over someone: to dominate.

To have time on one's hands: to have plenty of free time.

To keep one's hand in: to be in practice.

To lay hands on: to seize, touch (often used negatively).

To live from hand to mouth: to live from day to day; without regular money.

To play into someone's hands: to do something which helps one's opponent.

To rule with a heavy hand: to rule severely.

To say offhand: to give an answer immediately from memory.

To take one's courage in both hands: to force oneself to do something difficult, unpleasant.

To take someone in hand: to try to improve someone's behaviour.

To try one's hand at something: to make an attempt to do something new.

To wait on someone hand and foot: to attend to someone's needs with great care.

To wash one's hands of someone/something: to have nothing more to do with.

Head

A headache: a pain in the head; a difficult problem; a troublesome person.

From head to foot/toe: completely; all over the person.

It is on his head: he is responsible for it.

Not to know whether one is standing on one's head or one's heels: to be in a state of extreme confusion.

To be above/over one's head: too difficult to understand.

To be big-headed: to be conceited.

To be block-headed: to be dull, stupid.

To be fat-headed: to be stupid.

To be hard-headed: to be practical, unsentimental.

To be head and shoulders above others: to be much taller; to be far better.

To be head over heels in love: completely, very much in love.

To be hot-headed: to be hasty, impulsive.

To be pig-headed: to be obstinate.

To be soft-headed: to be simple-minded.

To be touched in the head: to be slightly mad.

To bite a person's head off: to speak sharply, angrily to someone.

To bury one's head in the sand: to avoid facing facts by pretending not to see them.

To come to a head: to reach a crisis.

To eat one's head off: to eat an excessive amount.

To get one's head down: to go to bed.

To get something into one's head: be convinced that something is true.

To go off one's head: to become crazy, mad.

To go to one's head: to make one excited, to intoxicate one.

To have a good head for business: to have a natural aptitude for it.

To have a good head-piece: to have plenty of brains.

To have a head: to have a headache, often from drinking too much.

To have a head like a sieve: to be very forgetful.

To have an old head on young shoulders: to be wise beyond one's years.

To have one's head screwed on the right way: to be intelligent, full of common sense, especially in practical matters.

To have something hanging over one's head: to have some danger, something unpleasant going to happen soon.

To head off: to divert a person from someone or something.

To heap coals of fire on a person's head: to treat a person well who has treated oneself badly.

To hit the nail on the head: to guess right, to reach the correct conclusion.

To keep one's head: to stay calm in a difficult situation.

To keep one's head above water: to keep out of debt.

To knock on the head: to destroy, disrupt an idea, plan, etc.

To knock/run one's head against a stone wall: to do something that will fail, because of opposition.

To let someone have his head: to let him do as he wishes.

To lose one's head: to lose one's self-control in a difficult situation.

To make head, headway: to make progress.

To make head or tail of something: to understand it. (Usually used negatively, e.g. 'I couldn't make head or tail of the letter he sent me'.)

To put something out of one's head: to forget it deliberately, to stop thinking about it.

To put things into someone's head: to suggest things to him.

To take it into one's head: to make a sudden decision.

To talk someone's head off: to talk so much that the other person is weary.

Two heads are better than one: two people know more together than one person alone.

Heart

After one's own heart: a person sharing one's own interests, opinions.

At heart: basically, deep down.

Have a heart!: Be reasonable; don't be unkind!

Heartache: deep sorrow, grief.

Heartburn: pain in chest as a result of indigestion, pyrosis.

Heart-felt sympathy: deepest sympathy.

Heart-searching: doubts, uncertainties.

In one's heart of hearts: deep down in oneself.

Not to have the heart to do something: not to have the courage to do something.

The heart of the matter: the essence, the vital part.

To be downhearted: to be depressed.

To be good at heart: to be good basically.

To be half-hearted about something: not to be very enthusiastic.

To be hard-hearted: to be hard, unkind.

To be heartless: to be unkind, unsympathetic.

To be hearty: to be cheerful.

To be in good heart: to be cheerful, confident.

To be lion-hearted: to be very brave.

To be soft-hearted: to be kind, sympathetic.

To be stout-hearted: to be very brave.

To break one's heart: to be overwhelmed with sorrow.

To cause heartache: to cause suffering.

To cry one's heart out: to cry excessively.

To eat one's heart out: to fret, worry excessively.

To have a big heart: to be warm, generous.

To have a heart: to have trouble with one's heart.

To have a heart-to-heart talk with someone: to speak openly, hiding nothing.

To have a hearty appetite: to have a very good appetite.

To have no heart: to be hard, insensitive.

To have no heart for something: to have no enthusiasm for something.

To have one's heart in one's boots: to be depressed, to feel hopeless.

To have one's heart in one's mouth: to be very afraid.

To know/learn/ say by heart: to know/learn/say something word for word by memory.

To lose heart: to have no hope, to become discouraged. (Often used negatively, e.g. 'Don't lose heart: keep on hoping'.)

To lose one's heart: to fall in love.

To put one's heart into something: to do something with enthusiasm.

To set one's heart on something: to want something very much.

To take heart: to become more hopeful.

To take someone to one's heart: to feel deep affection for someone.

To take something to heart: to be upset; to worry too much about things.

To tear one's heartstrings: to hurt one very deeply.

Whole-hearted: complete, without doubts.

Heel(s)

A heel: a completely unreliable person.

An/one's Achilles heel: weak or vulnerable point, especially of character.

Not to know whether one is standing on one's head or one's heels: to be in a state of extreme confusion.

To be down at heel: poorly dressed and in a state of poverty.

To be head over heels in love: completely, very much.

To bring someone to heel: to put them under control.

To carry with the heels first: as a dead body.

To come on the heels of: to follow immediately.

To kick one's heels: to stand waiting idly, impatiently.

To leave to cool his heels: to make someone wait deliberately.

To show a clean pair of heels: to run away.
To take to one's heels: to run away.

Knee

To be knee-deep in something: deeply involved in.
To be on one's knees: to kneel, especially when praying; to be completely exhausted.
To bring someone to his knees: to make him submit, stop fighting.
To go down on one's knees to someone: to beg for something.
To have a knees-up: a very lively party.

Knuckles

To knuckle down to a job: to work as hard as one can.
To knuckle under: to accept defeat.
To rap someone's knuckles: to reprimand.

Lap (waist to knees of one sitting)

In the lap of the gods: uncertain future.
In the lap of luxury: in great comfort and luxury.

Leg

A blackleg: a person who continues working when others are on strike.
Not to have a leg to stand on: have no good reason to support one's argument.
The boot is on the other leg: the truth is the opposite of what one believes.
To be on one's last legs: to be close to death; utterly weary.
To find one's legs: to be able to stand and walk (usually after an illness).
To get one's sea legs: to become used to the movement of a ship.
To give someone a leg up: to help someone.

To pull someone's leg: to tease someone.

To show a leg: to get out of bed.

To stretch one's legs: to go for a walk.

To walk someone off his legs: to tire him out with walking.

Lip

Lip: impudence, saucy talk.

None of your lip!: 'Don't speak to me like that!'

Lip-language, -reading, -speaking: use of the movement of the lips to and by the deaf and dumb.

A word escapes one's lips: something is said without thought.

To bite one's lip: to hide emotion, to stop oneself from saying something.

To curl one's lip: to show scorn.

To hang on someone's lip: to listen with great care.

To have sealed lips: to be silent about something.

To keep a stiff upper lip: to bear troubles without showing emotion.

To lick one's lips: to show appreciation of food (or sometimes other things).

To pay lip service to principles, etc.: to say one believes in something but not to act accordingly.

Mind

Mind: memory, remembrance.

Mind-blowing: (of drugs, etc.) causing ecstasy, excitement; (of news) confusing, shattering.

Mind-boggling: astonishing, extraordinary; overwhelming.

Never mind: 'It doesn't matter; don't worry'.

To be not in one's right mind: to be mad.

To be out of one's mind: to be mad.

To bear something in mind: to remember.

To bend someone's mind: to influence the mind so that it is permanently affected.

To give someone a piece of one's mind: to speak openly and critically.

To go out of one's mind: to go mad, e.g. 'He went out of his mind in the end'; to be forgotten, e.g. 'I'm so sorry. It went out of my mind'.

To have a lot on one's mind: to be worried about many things.

To have presence of mind: to act and think quickly in emergencies.

To know one's own mind: to be definite about what one wants.

To make up one's mind: to decide.

To mind: (a) To be careful (used very often in orders): 'Mind the step' – be careful of the step; 'Mind the car' – get out of the way of the car. (b) To care (often used negatively): 'I don't mind what she does or says'. (c) To object (used mainly interrogatively and negatively): 'I don't mind going to hospital to have my baby'. Note the polite request: 'Would you mind' + -ing form of the verb: 'Would you mind lying on the bed?'. (d) To take care of: 'She had no one to mind the baby when she went to work'. Noun: a baby-minder.

To mind one's own business: not to interfere in the affairs of other people.

To mind one's p's and q's: to be careful what one says and does.

To mind out for: avoid.

To take a load/weight off someone's mind: give great relief.

Mouth

Mouth: impudent talk, rudeness.

To be down in the mouth: to be depressed.

To look as if butter would not melt in one's mouth: to look innocent, incapable of badness.

To make one's mouth water: to cause saliva to flow at the sight of food.

To put words into someone's mouth: to tell someone what to say.

To take the words out of someone's mouth: to say what someone was about to say.

Nail(s)

(Note: Several idioms are listed which refer to other meanings of the word 'nail' than the nail of the body. They have been included because they are all commonly used and you should be familiar with them.)

Nail-biting: causing anxiety or tension.

To be as hard as nails: to be very tough; merciless.

To be as right as nails: to be perfectly fit.

To fight tooth and nail: to fight fiercely, vigorously.

To hit the nail on the head: to say the right thing, to guess right.

To nail someone down: to make someone give a definite statement; details.

To pay on the nail: to pay at once.

To put a nail in one's coffin: to do something that will shorten one's life.

Neck

Neck: boldness, disrespect, impertinence.

Neck or nothing: desperately risking everything for success.

Stiff-necked: obstinate, proud, stubborn.

To be a pain in the neck: to be a nuisance and pest to someone.

To be up to the neck in debt, work: to be completely immersed in debt, work.

To break one's neck to do something: work extremely hard to do something.

To get it in the neck: to be severely punished.

To have the neck to do something: to be rude enough to do something.

To neck: to hug and kiss someone intimately.

To run neck and neck: to be level with someone in a competition.

To save one's neck: to save oneself from punishment.

To stick one's neck out: to act or speak in a way which exposes one to harm or criticism.

To talk out of the back of one's neck: to talk nonsense.

To throw someone out neck and crop: to throw someone out head first, bodily.

Nerve(s)

Nerve-racking: frightening, stressful.
Not to know what nerves are: to have a calm temperament.
To be a bundle of nerves: in a very nervous state.
To get on one's nerves: to annoy or irritate very much.
To have a fit of nerves: to be in a nervous state.
To have iron/steel nerves: not to be easily upset or frightened.
To have the nerve to do something: to be brave, to be impudent enough.
To lose one's nerve: to become frightened and unsure of oneself.
To nerve oneself to do something: to use all one's strength, mental and physical.
To strain every nerve: to make a great effort.
What a nerve!: What impudence!

Nose

To cut off one's nose to spite one's face: to do something in anger to hurt someone else which also hurts oneself.
To follow one's nose: to go straight on, to act on instinct.
To get up a person's nose: to annoy someone.
To have a good nose: to have a good sense of smell.
To keep one's nose to the grindstone: to work hard over a long period.
To lead someone by the nose: to make someone do anything one wishes.
To look down one's nose at someone: to regard someone as inferior.
To nose about: to look enquiringly everywhere.
To pay through the nose: to pay an excessive price.
To poke one's nose into something: to try to find out about people

and things which do not concern one.

To put someone's nose out of joint: to do something to irritate or upset someone.

To see no further than one's nose: not to be able to imagine the future or any situation other than the current one.

To speak through one's nose: to speak with a nasal sound (often as a result of adenoids).

To turn up one's nose: to show dislike or disapproval.

Palm

To grease someone's palm: to bribe him, offer money for information, etc.

To palm something off on someone: to sell something that is worthless or damaged.

Shoulder

A shoulder to cry on: someone who listens to one's problems with sympathy.

Shoulder to shoulder: with united effort.

Straight from the shoulder: a strong blow or strong criticism of someone.

To cold-shoulder someone: to ignore someone deliberately; treat coldly.

To have a chip on one's shoulder: to go around with a sense of grievance.

To have an old head on young shoulders: a young person who is wise beyond his age.

To have broad shoulders: to be strong; to be able to bear responsibility.

To put one's shoulder to the wheel: to make a great effort to do something.

To rub shoulders with: to mix with people.

To shoulder (a burden or the blame): to carry.

Skin

A skinflint: a mean, miserly person.

A skinhead: a member of a group of young people who have closely cut hair, strange clothes and are often violent.

Skin-deep (of beauty, emotion, wound): no deeper than the skin, not lasting, on the surface.

To be skin and bone: very thin.

To be thick-skinned: not to care what others say about one, insensitive.

To be thin-skinned: to be too sensitive to what others say.

To escape by the skin of one's teeth: to have a narrow escape.

To get under one's skin: to annoy intensely, to hold one's interest very much.

To jump out of one's skin: to be startled, frightened suddenly.

To keep one's eyes skinned: to be watchful.

To save one's skin: to avoid or escape from danger.

To skin: for a wound to be covered with new skin; to remove skin from something.

Skull

Thick-skulled: dull, stupid person.

To get something into one's skull: to understand and remember it.

Stomach

To have a strong stomach: ability not to feel nausea; can eat anything.

To have butterflies in the stomach: to have fluttery feelings in the stomach due to nervousness.

To stomach something: accept. (Usually in negative form, e.g. 'He cannot stomach her ways', meaning he cannot bear them.)

To turn one's stomach: cause nausea; cause someone to be disgusted.

Teeth – see Tooth

Throat

Cut-throat competition: fierce, intense struggle in business.
Throaty: guttural, spoken in the throat.
To cut one's own throat: to act in a way that harms oneself; to kill oneself.
To have a frog in one's throat: hoarseness or loss of voice.
To have a lump in one's throat: to feel choked with emotion so that one can hardly speak.
To have a throat: to have a sore throat.
To have words stick in one's throat: to be too embarrassed by something to be able to speak of it.
To jump down someone's throat: to speak angrily to someone.
To thrust something down someone's throat: to try to make someone accept one's own beliefs, views, etc.

Thumb

Thumbs up!: mark of victory, satisfaction.
To be under someone's thumb: to be dominated by someone.
To thumb a lift: to sign with the thumb to ask a motorist for a free lift.
To twiddle one's thumbs: to have to sit still and do nothing.

Toe(s)

From top to toe: from head to foot, completely.
To be on one's toes: to be ready for action, alert.
To step/tread on someone's toes: to annoy someone unwittingly (often by doing what they want to do).
To tiptoe: to walk on the tips of one's toes; to walk quietly.
To toe the line: to obey the rules, of a party, society, etc.
To turn up one's toes: to die.

Tongue

A slip of the tongue: a mistake made when speaking.

Tongue: language (e.g. one's mother tongue, meaning one's native language).

To be tongue-tied: to be too shy, too nervous to speak.

To have a dangerous tongue: to speak maliciously.

To have a long tongue: to be talkative.

To have a ready tongue: to speak easily, fluently.

To have something on the tip of one's tongue: to be about to say something and then forget it.

To hold one's tongue: to be silent.

To lose one's tongue: to be too shy to speak.

To put out one's tongue: grimace to mark displeasure; for doctor's inspection.

To speak with one's tongue in one's cheek: to say something that is not true in order to joke with someone.

To wag one's tongue: to talk indiscreetly, to gossip.

Tooth, teeth

In the teeth of evidence, opposition, wind, etc.: against it.

Teething troubles: difficulties in the first stages of something.

To be armed to the teeth: to be fully armed with many weapons.

To be fed up to the back teeth with something: to be bored by, tired of.

To be long in the tooth: to be old.

To cast something in someone's teeth: to blame him for it.

To cut a tooth: a new tooth begins to show above the gum (of babies and children).

To cut one's eye-teeth: to gain worldly wisdom, maturity.

To cut one's wisdom teeth: (as to cut one's eye-teeth).

To escape by the skin of one's teeth: to have a narrow escape.

To fight tooth and nail: to fight with all one's strength.

To get one's teeth into something: to make an enthusiastic start on a job, etc.

To have a sweet tooth: to enjoy eating sweet things.

To set one's teeth on edge: to cause an unpleasant feeling in the teeth; to cause disgust.

To show one's teeth: to become aggressive.

To take the bit between one's teeth: to reject the advice and control of others.

Phrasal verbs

8

INTRODUCTION

'Phrasal verb' is a name given to those combinations of verb plus preposition or adverbial particle from which we have now hundreds of phrases to describe everyday events and activities.

The most commonly used phrasal verbs are formed from the shortest and simplest verbs in the English language such as come, do, get, go, make, put, take, followed by words such as down, from, in, out, up, to. A phrasal verb consists of two (sometimes three) parts and it is essential to consider the parts together, for the combination often makes a different meaning. Some phrasal verbs have several meanings.

Those who study the English language as a second language have great difficulty in understanding and using phrasal verbs correctly. For this reason a whole chapter is given to them. It is quite impossible to follow everyday speech without a knowledge of phrasal verbs, because we use them in preference to more formal words. To take some examples: we talk about 'getting up' in the morning and 'putting on our clothes' rather than 'rising' and 'dressing'.

Nurses, doctors and other health workers must use language understood easily by their patients, so they ask, for example, 'When did the pain first come on?' meaning the onset of pain, or say 'I want you to cut down on fatty foods', meaning to reduce intake. The examples given here are mostly taken from healthcare situations and so will be invaluable to you.

BREAK

— **Break down:**

   i. *collapse mentally or physically, often due to stress.* Nurse Foster worked too many double shifts and eventually her health broke down.

   ii. *cry with grief, shock, etc.* If I talk about losing my baby, I break down.

   iii. *fail to work because of electrical, mechanical, etc., fault.* The cardiac imaging system has broken down.

   iv. *fail, discontinue.* Negotiations over the ambulance workers' pay dispute have broken down.

— **Break in:** *enter somewhere by force.* I could never sleep alone in the house after burglars broke in.

— **Break out:** *sudden start of disease, fire, violence, war.* Food poisoning broke out in the care home.

— **Break out in something:** *suddenly become covered in.* (a) Whenever I eat strawberries I break out in a rash. (b) I keep waking up and breaking out in a cold sweat.

— **Break through:** *make a major discovery or advance.* The pharmaceutical company hopes to break through with a new treatment for Alzheimer's disease.

— **Break up:** *deteriorate (of health).* He's breaking up under the strain of nursing his wife.

— **Break something up:** *come to end (of relationships).* I've been ill ever since my marriage broke up.

— **Break with:** *end relations with someone.* My son has broken with us since he mixed with this group.

BRING

— **Bring something about:** *cause something to happen.* Drug misuse brought about his death.

— **Bring something back:** *call to mind.* Talking to you brings back memories of my childhood.

— **Bring someone back to something:** *restore.* A complete change will bring you back to health.

— **Bring someone down:** *defeat, degrade*. Heavy drinking brought him down.

— **Bring something down:** *lower, reduce*. Reducing your weight will help to bring down the cholesterol levels in your blood.

— **Bring something on:** *cause*. It would help me to know what brings on your chest pain.

— **Bring someone round:** *restore to consciousness*. The patient was brought round by mouth-to-mouth ventilation.

— **Bring someone through:** *save someone's life*. Her husband was critically ill but the doctors and nurses struggled all night to bring him through and he survived.

— **Bring someone to:** *restore to consciousness*.

— **Bring someone up:** *rear, teach a child social habits* (often used in the passive). His mother died when he was two so he was brought up by his grandmother. (*Note:* To be well brought up. To be badly brought up.)

— **Bring something up:**
   i. *vomit*. She's not well. She brought up her lunch today.
   ii. *eructation*. Do you bring any wind up?

COME

— **Come about:** *happen*. How did the accident come about? He slipped on a wet floor.

— **Come across:** *make an impression of a particular kind*. She comes across as a very nervous woman.

— **Come across someone/something:** *find, meet or see unexpectedly*. I've never come across such a bad case of shingles before.

— **Come along:** *make progress*. You're coming along nicely. We shall have you walking without crutches next week.

— **Come back:** *return*. (a) Make an appointment to come back in a month. (b) The stress symptoms have come back since I went back to work.

— **Come back to someone:** *return to memory*. Yes, what happened is all coming back to me now. I remember falling down the steps.

— **Come by something:** *get, obtain.* How did you come by that scar on your cheek? I was in a fight and someone threw a bottle at me.

— **Come down (of prices, temperature, etc.):** *be lowered, fall.* Your blood pressure has come down since we started you on the tablets.

— **Come down on someone:** *criticise someone, punish.* The police come down heavily on people found with class A drugs.

— **Come down with something:** *become ill with something.* She came down with flu and was unable to keep her appointment.

— **Come forward:** *present oneself, with help, information, etc.* Will anyone who saw the accident please come forward?

— **Come from:** *have as one's birthplace* (not used in the continuous tenses). Where do you come from? I come from India.

— **Come in:**

   i. *be admitted to hospital.* We'd like your mother to come in so we can do one or two tests.

   ii. *be introduced, begin to be used.* More people were treated quicker and better when day surgery and keyhole surgery came in.

— **Come off something:** *fall from a bicycle, horse, etc.* My son came off his motor bike and broke his left leg.

— **Come on:**

   i. *encourage someone to hurry, make an effort, try harder* (used in imperative only). Come on Mr Hopkins. Let's see you walk across the room now.

   ii. *grow, make progress.* Good. Your baby's coming on very well.

   iii. *start (of symptoms, etc.)* Tell me exactly when these panic attacks first came on.

— **Come out:**

   i. *be published.* When's your new book coming out?

   ii. *become known.* It's just come out that they are closing down the factory and I shall lose my job.

iii. *publicly acknowledge one's homosexuality*. John and Simon have come out.

iv. *stop work, strike*. Do you think health professionals should come out for better working conditions?

— **Come out in something:** *be partially covered in rash, spots, etc*. Her hands came out in a rash after she used a new detergent.

— **Come over:** *begin to feel dizzy, faint, etc*. It's happened twice now travelling home from work. I came over faint.

— **Come round:** *regain consciousness*. Your son hasn't come round yet from the anaesthetic.

— **Come through something:** *recover from a serious illness, accident, survive*. You're lucky to have come through such a terrible accident.

— **Come to:** *regain consciousness*. When I came to, I was on the bathroom floor.

— **Come under something:** *be classified as*. Diamorphine and cocaine come under Class A of the Misuse of Drugs Act.

— **Come up:**

i. *arise (of a subject)*. The question of the rights of patients is always coming up these days.

ii. *happen, occur*. I'm afraid I shall be late for my clinic. Something urgent has come up.

CUT

— **Cut back (on) something:** *reduce expenditure*. Because of financial restrictions, all departments have had to cut back drastically.

— **Cut something down; cut down (on something):** *reduce amount or quantity*. (a) I've already cut my cigarettes down to 10 a day. (b) You should cut down on the fats you eat.

— **Cut someone off:** *break the connection on the telephone* (often used in passive). How annoying. I've just been cut off in the middle of a conversation.

— **Cut something off:**
   i. *amputate, remove.* Following the explosion, the man had to have his left leg cut off.
   ii. *stop the supply of something* (often used in passive). The electricity has been cut off.
— **Cut off:** *isolated.* She feels very cut off since she got cancer.
— **Cut out something:**
   i. *excise.* I had a lump on my neck cut out.
   ii. *stop eating, using.* I've cut out alcohol completely.
— **Cut someone up:** *upset emotionally* (usually in the passive). He was terribly cut up by his wife's death.

DO

— **Do away with oneself:** *to commit suicide, kill oneself.* I feel so depressed, Nurse. I could do away with myself.
— **Do someone in:**
   i. *exhaust* (usually in passive). At the end of the week I'm absolutely done in.
   ii. *kill* (usually in passive). The old man was done in (slang).
— **Do something in:** *injure a part of the body.* He did his back in moving furniture.
— **Do something to something:** *cause something to happen* (questions often start with *what*). What have you done to your leg? It's bleeding.
— **Do something up:**
   i. *fasten with buttons or zip, etc.* Well, Mr Cox, let's see if you can do up your clothes.
   ii. *modernise, redecorate, restore.* These wards are depressing. They need doing up.
— **Do with something:**
   i. *be concerned with, connected with* (use with *have to*). His job has something to do with nursing research.
   ii. *need, wish for* (used with *can* and *could*). You could do with some new glasses. Go and have your eyes tested.
— **Do without someone/something:** *manage without.* We've

had to do without a speech and language therapist since the last one left.

FIND

— **Find something out:** *discover the truth, learn some information.* When did you find out your son was on drugs?

FIT

— **Fit someone/something in:** *manage to find time to see someone or do something.* The nurse is booked up all morning, but as it's urgent I'll try and fit you in.
— **Fit in with someone/something:** *suit, harmonise with someone/something.* Do you think she will fit in with the rest of the team?
— **Fit someone/something out/up with:** *equip.* After the operation, we'll fit you up with a seat to get you into the bath.

GET

— **Get about:**
   i. *move from place to place.* I can't get about much now that I've got arthritis.
   ii. *spread (of news, rumour).* It got about that the Community Hospital might close.
— **Get something across:** *communicate something to someone.* It's quite difficult to get across to my mother that she can't go on living alone.
— **Get along:** *make progress.* Fine. You're getting along very well.
— **Get along with someone:** *have a good relationship with somebody.* Do you get along with your family?
— **Get around:** — as for *Get about.*
— **Get at someone:** *criticise someone repeatedly* (usually in continuous tenses). The other children are always getting at him

and he's afraid of going to school now.

— **Get at someone/something:**

   i. *reach*. Make sure you put these tablets somewhere where the children can't get at them.

   ii. *mean, try to say*. I'm not sure what you're getting at.

— **Get away:** *have a holiday*. You should try to get away for a few days after the operation.

— **Get back:** *arrive, return home*. He says he can get back under his own steam (without help).

— **Get back to someone:** *contact someone again later*. I don't have the information you need just now, but I'll get back to you.

— **Get something back:** *recover something that was lost*. He's now got back the use of his arm which was paralysed by the stroke.

— **Get by:** *manage, cope with life*. Lone-parent families often have a struggle to get by.

— **Get someone down:** *depress*. All this quarrelling in the family gets me down.

— **Get something down:** *swallow* (with difficulty). The tablets you gave me last time were so big I could hardly get them down.

— **Get into:** *start bad habits*. How did she get into drugs?

— **Get (someone) off:** *fall asleep, help someone to fall asleep*. It takes me ages to get the baby off at night.

— **Get off something:** *leave work with permission*. He got a week off when his wife had a baby.

— **Get on:**

   i. *perform* (often used in questions with *how*). (a) How did you get on in the exam? (b) I got on fine with my first assignment but failed my second.

   ii. *progress*. Take these tablets for a month and we'll see how you get on.

— **Get on with someone:** *have a good relationship with*. I get on fine with my children, but I don't get on with my wife.

— **Get out:** *leave the house*. You must try to get out more. No wonder you are depressed, sitting here alone all day.

— **Get out of something:**
   i. *escape the necessity or duty to do something*. He managed to get out of working nights for a month.
   ii. *give up a habit*. I wish I could get out of the habit of smoking after every meal.

— **Get over something:**
   i. *overcome*. No need to worry. I'm sure we can get over that problem.
   ii. *recover from disappointment, illness, shock*. He's getting over the shock of losing his wife extremely well.

— **Get something over:** *complete something difficult or unpleasant*. Thank goodness I've got the hysterectomy over.

— **Get something over to someone:** *make someone understand*. You must get over to your husband the importance of remaining active as far as possible.

— **Get through something:**
   i. *consume, use a certain amount*. He gets through a bottle of spirits a day.
   ii. *pass an exam, test*. Marvellous. I've got through my driving test.

— **Get through to someone:**
   i. *make contact, communicate*. We are in despair. We just can't get through to our son at all.
   ii. *reach, especially by telephone*. I've tried six times to speak to the stoma care nurse, but I can't get through.

— **Get together:** *assemble, meet*. The management and the union should get together to settle this problem.

— **Get up:** *rise from bed*. Do you have to get up in the night to pass water?

— **Get up to something:** *do something surprising or unacceptable*. My parents have no idea what I get up to.

GIVE

— **Give something back to someone:** *restore, return*. The operation should give you back the use of your legs.

— **Give in (to someone/something):** *stop arguing, fighting, trying, etc.* Mrs Spearey was marvellous. She had so much illness but she would not give in.

— **Give out:**
  i. *come to an end* (of food supplies, strength, etc.). I can't go on any longer. My strength has given out.
  ii. *fail, stop working.* At the end of the 6-hour operation, the patient's heart gave out and he died.

— **Give something out:** *distribute.* Those leaflets must be given out to all staff explaining the new safety regulations.

— **Give someone up:**
  i. *renounce hope.* The doctors had given her up months ago, but she made a marvellous recovery.
  ii. *stop having a relationship with someone.* Why don't you give him up if he treats you so badly?

— **Give something up:** *stop doing something.* (a) How can I give up smoking? (b) I used to be a teacher, but I gave it up last year.

GO

— **Go against something:** *conflict with something.* Private medicine goes against the principles of the NHS set up in 1948.

— **Go ahead with something:** *proceed with something.* I've decided I want to go ahead with the job application.

— **Go along with someone/something:**
  i. *accompany.* Nurse, go along with Mrs Hooper to the X-Ray Department, will you?
  ii. *agree.* I can't go along with your idea of a further operation.

— **Go at someone:** *attack physically or verbally.* I was walking down the street and a young man went at me, knocked me to the ground and took my bag.

— **Go back:** *return.* I want you to go back to your GP with this letter.

— **Go by:** *pass (of time).* As time goes by, you'll get more used to wearing the artificial limb.

— **Go by something:** *form an opinion.* I know I look well, but that's nothing to go by. I feel terrible.

— **Go down:**

   i. *be swallowed* (of food and drink). My food won't go down (i.e. I have difficulty swallowing food).

   ii. *be reduced in size, level, etc.* How's your ankle? Well, the swelling has gone down, but it's still very painful.

   iii. *become lower, fall* (of prices, temperature, weight, etc.) (a) His temperature has gone down. (b) I used to be 9 stone 7 pounds, but then I lost my appetite and went down to 8½ stones.

   iv. *decrease in quality, deteriorate.* Standards of behaviour have gone down in recent years.

— **Go down with something:** *become ill with something.* All the children have gone down with measles.

— **Go for someone:** *attack physically or verbally.* He went for her with a knife.

— **Go for someone/something:** *Fetch.* Go for Sister, quickly.

— **Go in for:**

   i. *enter for an examination.* Thousands of nurses go in for higher degrees every year.

   ii. *study for a particular profession.* Are you going in for medicine like your mother?

— **Go into something:** *investigate.* The Neonatal Intensive Care Unit has been closed while the authorities go into the sudden deaths of ten babies.

— **Go off:**

   i. *deteriorate, get worse.* Her work has gone off since the accident.

   ii. *explode.* She had to have plastic surgery after an oil heater went off in her face.

   iii. *faint, fall asleep, lose consciousness.* (a) If he sees blood, he goes off. (b) It takes me ages to go off. Sometimes I take a sleeping pill.

   iv. *go bad* (of food or drink), *become unfit to eat or drink.*

The food poisoning was caused by eating some meat that had gone off.

v. *stop* (of pain). I've had this abdominal pain for a month. When I take the tablets it goes off, but it comes back.

— **Go off someone/something:** *to lose one's liking or taste for someone/something.* (a) My wife's gone off me. (Usually means does not wish to continue sexual relationship.) (b) I've gone off drink since my operation. (c) I've gone off my food completely.

— **Go on:**

i. *continue.* (a) This trouble with your bowels has been going on for years, hasn't it? (When followed by a verb, the verb is in the -ing form.) (b) Go on taking the tablets. (c) Should I go on working while I'm pregnant, Sister? It is often used negatively: (d) I can't go on any longer like this. Can you give me something to help me, Nurse?

ii. *happen, take place.* What's going on?

— **Go on something:**

i. *begin to receive payments from the State because of unemployment.* We've had to go on Social Security as we've no other money coming in.

ii. *go on the pill; begin to take the contraceptive pill.* When did you first go on the pill?

— **Go on at someone:** *to complain of someone's behaviour, work, etc.* He never stops going on at me.

— **Go out:**

i. *be extinguished* (of fire, light, etc.). All the lights have gone out.

ii. *leave the house.* (a) I'm longing to go out again. (b) You should be able to go out in a couple of days.

— **Go over something:** *check, inspect details, repeat.* Well, I've told you what the treatment involves and I'm going to go over it again to make sure you understand.

— **Go round:** *spread from person to person* (of illness). There's a nasty virus going round at the moment.

— **Go round to:** *pay a visit locally.* I went round to see the practice nurse last week and he sent me here.

— **Go through:** *endure, experience, suffer.* (a) When did he go through the phase of passing loose stools? (b) She's gone through a very bad patch recently (an unhappy or difficult time). (c) I can't tell you what I've gone through since my husband died.

— **Go under:**

   i. *have an anaesthetic.* The patient went under at 12 and came round at 4 o'clock.

   ii. *die* (slang). Do you think he's going to go under?

— **Go up:** *rise* (of blood pressure, temperature, etc.). Your blood pressure has gone up again.

— **Go with someone:** *accompany.* Have you anyone who can go with you to hospital?

— **Go without something:** *manage without something.* (a) I have to go without food before I have the barium enema. (b) They went without sleep for several days.

KEEP

— **Keep away from someone/something:** *avoid being near to.* Keep away from anyone with German measles if you think you are pregnant.

— **Keep someone/something back:** *hold back.* (a) My disability will never keep me back. (b) She couldn't keep back her tears.

— **Keep someone down:** *dominate, oppress.* They had a difficult childhood. Their father kept them down.

— **Keep something down:**

   i. *keep something in the stomach* (often used negatively meaning to vomit). She's so thin because she can't keep anything down.

   ii. *not increase something* (e.g. wages, prices, weight, etc.). (a) Keep your weight down. (b) Restricting salt in the diet may help keep blood pressure down.

— **Keep someone from doing something:** *prevent.* All this coughing keeps me from sleeping.

— **Keep off something:** *not drink, eat, smoke, etc.* (a) Keep off fatty foods. (b) You should keep off alcohol while you're taking these tablets.

— **Keep on doing something:** *continue doing something, do something repeatedly.* The majority of women in the UK keep on working nowadays. (*Note:* 'keep doing something' has the same meaning as 'keep on doing something'.) Michael keeps getting stomach cramps.

— **Keep to something:** *adhere to an agreement, a course, a diet, etc.* Keep to the diet for another 2 months and then we'll see how you are.

— **Keep someone up:** *prevent someone from going to bed.* The baby kept us up all night with his crying.

— **Keep one's spirits, strength up:** *not allow to fall.* (a) She is a very brave woman and always keeps her spirits up. (Remains cheerful.) (b) You must eat to keep your strength up.

— **Keep up with someone/something:** *move, progress at the same rate.* Older people find it difficult to keep up with all the changes of modern life.

LET

— **Let someone down:** *disappoint, fail to help.* I can't leave the course. I can't let my parents down.

— **Let up:**

i. *become less intense, severe.* If only this pain would let up for a while.

ii. *relax one's efforts.* After the train crash, the team at the hospital worked night and day to treat the injured. Finally, they were able to let up a little.

LOOK

— **Look after oneself/someone:** *take care of.* (a) She is old and frail and needs to be properly looked after. (b) Who will look after your children when you come into hospital?

— **Look after something:** *be responsible for.* The technicians look after the equipment and keep it in good order.

— **Look at something:** *examine carefully.* I want to look at your ear to see what's causing the trouble.

— **Look down on someone/something:** *feel superior.* Her husband looks down on her because she hasn't been to university.

— **Look forward to doing something:** *think of something in the future with pleasure.* I'm looking forward to having this plaster cast off.

— **Look in:** *make a short visit to someone's house.* The social worker will look in again next week.

— **Look into something:** *investigate.* We must look into this complaint. It says someone was left lying on a trolley in the corridor for several hours without being attended to.

— **Look on:** *watch something without taking part.* Whilst the surgeon performed the delicate operation, doctors from many countries looked on.

— **Look on someone/something:** *consider.* He's looked on as one of the leading nurses in this field.

— **Look out:** *be careful, watch out.* Look out! You'll burn yourself on that stove.

— **Look out for someone/something:** *watch carefully for someone/something.* When assessing people, nurses look out for signs that indicate a problem.

— **Look over:** *inspect buildings, papers, etc.* Can you look over this report before I submit it to the Working Party?

— **Look through something:** *examine papers quickly.* I'll just look through the notes before seeing Ms Turner.

— **Look to someone/something:** *take care of.* The child-minder looks to the children while I'm at work.

— **Look up:**
   i. *improve.* How's Mrs Cox? Oh, she's looking up.
   ii. *raise eyes.* Open your eyes now and look up. I'm going to put some drops in your eyes.

— **Look someone up:** *visit someone, especially after a long time apart.* Do look me up when you next come to Birmingham.

— **Look something up:** *search for a word, fact in a reference book.* If you don't understand the colloquial English your patient uses, look it up in the Manual.

— **Look up to someone:** *admire, respect.* Young boys like to look up to pop stars and footballers.

MAKE

— **Make something of someone/something:** *understand the nature or meaning of someone/something.* (a) We don't know what to make of this change in her behaviour. (b) What do you make of it all?

— **Make off with something:** *to steal something and run away with it.* The youth made off with the CDs he'd found.

— **Make someone out:** *understand someone's behaviour.* We just can't make Mary out at all. She's changed so much since she left home.

— **Make something out:**
   i. *manage to read.* Can you make out what this letter says?
   ii. *manage to understand.* We'll have to get an interpreter. We just can't make out what this person says.
   iii. *write a cheque, a prescription, etc.* The nurse specialist made out a prescription for my asthma.

— **Make up:** *apply cosmetics.* Whenever I make up, I come out in a rash all over my face.

— **Make something up:**
   i. *invent a story, especially to deceive someone.* Stop making things up. What really happened?
   ii. *prepare a bed.* Keep Mr Derby here. The bed hasn't been made up yet.
   iii. *prepare medicine.* Take this prescription to the pharmacist and he'll make it up for you.
   iv. *supply deficiency.* It's not harmful to be a blood donor. The loss of blood is made up quite quickly in a healthy person.

— **Make up for something:** *compensate.* No amount of money can make up for the loss of her husband.

PUT

— **Put something aside:** *save money, etc., for future use.* Everything costs so much these days. I can't put anything aside for my old age.

— **Put someone away:** *to confine someone to prison or psychiatric unit* (often used in passive). (a) The old man began to wander in the street at night so his family put him away. (b) He was put away for life for murder.

— **Put something away:** *save money for future use.*

— **Put something back:**
  i. *drink large amount of alcohol* (slang). He must have put back a lot of beer to be in this state.
  ii. *impede.* The accident has put back his hopes of running in the Olympics.

— **Put something by:** *save money for future use.* Have you anything put by?

— **Put something down:**
  i. *kill animal because it is suffering or sick.* I had to have my dog put down last week.
  ii. *place a baby in bed.* I put him down at 9 and he starts crying at 11.
  iii. *write down.* I'd better put down when to take the tablets or I shall forget.

— **Put something down to:** *consider something is caused by.* What do you put this rash down to, Nurse? I put it down to an allergy.

— **Put something forward:** *propose, suggest.* At the meeting it was put forward that more operations should be dealt with in the Day Surgery Unit.

— **Put something in:**
  i. *install.* We aim to put strategies in that will reduce deaths from cancers by at least a fifth in people under 75 years by 2010.
  ii. *spend time on work.* Health professionals often put in many extra hours at work.

— **Put in for something:** *apply for a job.* He's put in for over 20

G-grade jobs without any success.

— **Put someone off (something):** *disturb, upset.* (a) She could never be a nurse. She's easily put off by the sight of blood. (b) Food just puts me off at the moment.

— **Put someone off doing something:** *dissuade someone from doing something.* My parents tried to put me off living with Tom, but I took no notice.

— **Put something off:** *delay, postpone.* The operation had to be put off because there was no bed available in the ICU.

— **Put something on:**
   i. *get dressed.* You can put your clothes on now, Mrs Turner.
   ii. *increase weight.* Good. You've put on 6 pounds since we last saw you.

   Put someone out:
   i. *anaesthetise.* They put me out and I came round 3 hours later (slang).
   ii. *annoy, upset.* She was put out because her doctor didn't explain what the procedure involved.

— **Put something out:**
   i. *dislocate.* I think you've put your shoulder out and we must X-ray it to be sure.
   ii. *extinguish fire, light.* Fire crews soon put the fire out.

— **Put someone through:** *connect on telephone.* Put me through to A&E will you please?

— **Put someone up:** *provide a bed and food.* I lost my job and my home. A friend put me up for a few weeks, but I'm homeless again.

— **Put something up:**
   i. *increase price.* My landlord has put the rent up by £20 a week so I'll have to go.
   ii. *raise.* The pain's so bad I can't put my arms up to do my hair.

— **Put up with someone/something:** *bear, tolerate.* (a) I'm afraid there's not much they can do about this condition. I'll have to put up with it. (b) How did she put up with that violent husband for so long?

RUN

— **Run across someone/something:** *to meet someone or find something by chance*. I've never run across this before. I think it's a case of botulism.

— **Run away from someone/something:** *suddenly leave, escape*. He's always been a difficult child. He ran away from home at the age of 10.

— **Run someone/something down:**
  i. *hit and knock to the ground*. The cyclist was run down by a lorry.
  ii. *speak badly about someone*. He's always running down his girlfriend in public.

— **Run someone in:** *arrest and take to police station*. He was run in for shoplifting (slang).

— **Run into something:**
  i. *collide or crash into*. A man has just been brought into A&E. He ran his car into a wall in the fog.
  ii. *get into danger, debt, trouble, etc*. We've run into debt and my partner's drinking heavily.

— **Run something off:** *make copies on a machine*. Could you run off 20 copies of this hand-out, please?

— **Run out of something:** *come to an end* (of permits, supplies, time, etc.). (a) Make sure we've enough clean sheets this weekend. We mustn't run out. (b) I'm nearly 85 you know. I'm running out of time. (c) My energy is running out.

— **Run over someone:** (of a vehicle) *knock someone down and pass over body*. He's been run over and has multiple injuries.

— **Run over something:** *read quickly, repeat*. Will you just run over the facts again?

— **Run through something:**
  i. *discuss, examine, read quickly*. I've run through the names of people admitted this week, but your son's is not there.
  ii. *spend carelessly, wastefully* They have run through thousands of pounds on advertising.

iii. *use up*. We run through a lot of disposable gloves in the sexual health clinic.

— **Run up something:** *accumulate bills*. Why did you run up such large bills?

SEND

— **Send for someone:** *tell someone to come*. He's failing. Send for the ambulance.
— **Send for something:** *order something to be delivered*. Send for the latest information, will you please?
— **Send off something:** *post*. Don't forget to send off those letters today.

SET

— **Set aside something:**
   i. *save money for particular purpose*. She sets aside a bit of money every month to pay her fuel bills.
   ii. *keep time for a particular purpose*. You must set aside half an hour a day to practise the relaxation exercises.
— **Set back someone/something:** *delay progress of someone/ something*. (a) Mr Deakin was making a good recovery after his operation, but unfortunately a wound infection has set him back. (b) Work on the new theatre has been set back 3 months.
— **Set in:** *begin and seem likely to continue* (of infection, rain, winter, etc.). (a) When cold weather sets in, older people must take precautions to care for themselves. (b) You can see gangrene has set in to your left leg and, as it has not responded to treatment, we have no alternative but to remove it.
— **Set on someone:** *attack*. I got this bite when a dog set on me.
— **Set someone up:** *make better, healthier*. A week by the sea will set you up after the bowel surgery.

TAKE

— **Take after someone:** *resemble in appearance or character*.

I'm worried about Jane. She's so different from me. She takes after her father.

— **Take something away:**

i. *cause a feeling, etc., to disappear.* (a) I'll give you some tablets to take the pain away. (b) All this worry has taken my appetite away.

ii. *remove.* They've taken her womb away.

— **Take someone away from someone/something:** *remove.* When sexual abuse was suspected, the children were taken away from their parents on the recommendation of social workers.

— **Take something down:** *record, write something.* Can you take down the details?

— **Take something in:** *absorb, understand by listening or reading.* He was so confused he could not take in what the nurse was saying.

— **Take something off:**

i. *amputate part of body.* His left arm had to be taken off below the elbow.

ii. *have time away from work for special purpose.* I'm taking next week off to be at home when my wife comes out of hospital.

iii. *lose weight by dieting.* I'm overweight. I want to take off a stone.

iv. *remove part of clothing.* You needn't take off all your clothes. Just your shirt.

— **Take on something:** *agree to do work, have responsibility.* Don't take on too much for the next 6 weeks.

— **Take something out:** *remove or extract.* (a) I must have this tooth taken out. It's giving me a lot of pain. (b) She's going into hospital to have her appendix taken out. (c) We're going to take the stitches out tomorrow.

— **Take something over from someone:** *take control, responsibility from someone else.* Can you take over my bleep for 10 minutes while I see Mrs Briggs?

— **Take to someone:** *develop a liking for someone.* I never took to my daughter-in-law. She's caused so much trouble in the family.

— **Take to something/doing something:** *begin to do something as a habit*. (a) We need help. Our only daughter has taken to drugs. (b) He's taken to going for long walks late at night.

— **Take up something:**

i. *absorb, occupy time*. Nursing takes up all his time and energy.

ii. *start a job*. We expect you to take up your duties on 1st January.

iii. *start a profession, hobby, etc*. He's thinking of taking up mental health nursing as a career.

TURN

— **Turn against someone:** *become hostile to*. After our divorce, my wife tried to turn the children against me.

— **Turn someone away:** *refuse to give help*. Health professionals cannot turn sick people away.

— **Turn someone/something down:**

i. *reject an idea, person, proposal*. They turned me down as a pilot because of my eyesight.

ii. *reduce volume of gas, sound, etc*. When they turn down the television I can't hear a thing.

— **Turn in:**

i. *go to bed* (slang). It's usually 2 o'clock before I turn in.

ii. *be pigeon-toed*. He walks with his toes turned in.

— **Turn something in:** *stop doing something* (slang). The job was ruining my health so, although I loved it, I had to turn it in.

— **Turn someone off:** *cause someone to be disgusted by something or not sexually attracted to someone*. His drinking and bad breath turned me off.

— **Turn something off:**

i. *stop the flow of electricity, gas, etc*. Don't forget to turn off the machine before you leave the building.

ii. *stop radio, TV.* The TV is going all day. He never turns it off.

— **Turn on someone:** *attack.* As I left the building, the guard dog turned on me and bit my leg.

— **Turn someone on:** *give great pleasure, excite sexually.* Certain illicit drugs turn you on very quickly.

— **Turn something on:** *allow gas, electricity, water to flow.* Make sure the computer is turned on first thing.

— **Turn someone out:** *force someone to leave a place.* I've nowhere to sleep. My partner has turned me out.

— **Turn something out:** *extinguish light or fire.* Please turn out the lights before going home.

— **Turn out:** *prove to be.* I never thought it would turn out to be fatal.

— **Turn over:** *change position of body by rolling.* Turn over onto your left side and draw your knees to your chest.

— **Turn someone/something round:** *face in different direction.* Turn round and let me look at your back.

— **Turn to someone/something:** *go for advice, help.* (a) The practice nurse is a good person to turn to when you need health advice. (b) Sadly, when his wife left him he turned to drink for solace.

— **Turn up:**
   i. *appear, arrive.* Mr Fox hasn't turned up yet for his appointment.
   ii. *be found, by chance, after being lost.* Thank goodness those keys have turned up. We thought they'd been stolen.

— **Turn something up:** *increase volume of radio, TV, etc.* I have to turn up my hearing aid to listen to the news.

Abbreviations used in nursing

9

INTRODUCTION

The rapid developments in nursing, healthcare and the related sciences in recent years have brought a vast increase in the associated vocabulary. At the same time, the increased speed of life has driven people to use abbreviations more and more, and this tendency is well illustrated in the nursing and healthcare field.

The use of abbreviations is discouraged because they are variable and misleading. The same initials may have different meanings in different areas of nursing practice. For example, PID may mean *pelvic inflammatory disease* or *prolapsed intervertebral disc*. The Nursing and Midwifery Council is clear about the need to avoid the use of abbreviations in record keeping and documentation (NMC 2002) (see Ch. 4).

Nevertheless, you will see and hear abbreviations being used every day in medical reports and notes and in discussions about patients and during handover reports, and a knowledge of them is, therefore, absolutely essential. You should always ask if you are not sure what an abbreviation means.

A selection of abbreviations commonly used by nurses and other health professionals is provided to help you understand what people mean.

A

AA – Alcoholics Anonymous

AAA – abdominal aortic aneurysm

ABG – arterial blood gas

a.c. – ante cibum (Latin – sometimes used in prescriptions), before food

ACE – angiotensin-converting enzyme

ACTH – adrenocorticotrophic hormone

ADH – antidiuretic hormone

ADHD – attention-deficit hyperactivity disorder

ad lib – ad libitum (Latin), to the desired amount

ADLs – Activities of Daily Living

ADRs – adverse drug reactions

A&E – Accident and Emergency Department

AF – atrial fibrillation

AFB – acid-fast bacilli

AFP – α-fetoprotein

AI – artificial insemination

AIDS – acquired immune deficiency syndrome

ALL – acute lymphoblastic leukaemia

ALs – Activities of Living

ALS – advanced life support

ALT – alanine aminotransferase

AMI – acute myocardial infarction

AML – acute myeloid leukaemia

ANC – antenatal care

ANS – autonomic nervous system

AP – anteroposterior

APEL – accreditation of prior experience and learning.

APH – antepartum haemorrhage

APKD – adult polycystic kidney disease

ARC – AIDS-related complex

ARDS – adult respiratory distress syndrome

ARF – (1) acute renal failure; (2) acute respiratory failure

ASD – atrial septal defect

AST – aspartate aminotransferase

ATN – acute tubular necrosis

ATD – Alzheimer's-type dementia

A-V – atrioventricular: (1) node; (2) bundle

B

BAI – Beck Anxiety Inventory

BAN – British Approved Name (of drugs)

BBA – born before arrival

BBB – (1) blood–brain barrier; (2) bundle branch block

BBVs – blood-borne viruses

BCG – bacille Calmette Guérin

b.d. – bis die (Latin – sometimes used in prescriptions), twice daily

BDI – Beck Depression Inventory

BHS – Beck Hopelessness Scale

b.i.d. – bis in die (Latin), twice a day

BID – brought in dead

BLS – basic life support

BMI – body mass index

BMR – basal metabolic rate

BMT – bone marrow transplant

BN – Bachelor of Nursing

BNF – *British National Formulary*

BNO – bowels not opened

BO – bowels opened

BP – (1) blood pressure; (2) *British Pharmacopoeia*

BPH – benign prostatic hyperplasia

BPRS – Brief Psychiatric Rating Scale

BSA – body surface area

BSc – Bachelor of Science

BSc (Soc Sc-Nurs) – Bachelor of Science (Nursing)

BSE – (1) bovine spongiform encephalopathy; (2) breast self-examination

BSS – Beck Scale for Suicide Ideation

B Wt – birth weight

C

C – (1) carbon; (2) centigrade (temperature scale)

Ca – carcinoma

CABG – coronary artery bypass grafting

CAN – Camberwell Assessment of Need

CAPD – continuous ambulatory peritoneal dialysis

CAPE – Clifton Assessment Procedures for the Elderly

CATS – credit accumulation transfer scheme

cc – cubic centimetre

CCF – congestive cardiac failure

CCU – Coronary Care Unit

CD – controlled drug

CDC – Centers for Disease Control and Prevention

CDS – Calgary Depression Scale

CEA – carcinoembryonic antigen

CF – (1) cardiac failure; (2) cystic fibrosis

CHAI – Commission for Healthcare Audit and Inspection

CHD – (1) congenital heart disease; (2) coronary heart disease

CHF – congestive heart failure

CIN – cervical intraepithelial neoplasia

CINAHL – Cumulative Index to Nursing and Allied Health Literature

CJD – Creutzfeldt–Jakob disease

CK – creatine kinase

CLL – chronic lymphatic leukaemia

cm – centimetre

CML – chronic myeloid leukaemia

CMV – cytomegalovirus

CNS – (1) central nervous system; (2) clinical nurse specialist

C/O – complains of

COPD – chronic obstructive pulmonary disease

COSHH – Control of Substances Hazardous to Health

CPA – care programme approach

CPAP – continuous positive airways pressure

CPD – continuing professional development

CPN – community psychiatric nurse

CPR – cardiopulmonary resuscitation

CRF – chronic renal failure

CSCI – Commission for Social Care Inspection

CSF – (1) cerebrospinal fluid; (2) colony stimulating factor

CSI – Caregiver Strain Index

CSSD – Central Sterile Supply Department

CSU – catheter specimen of urine

CT – (1) computed tomography; (2) coronary thrombosis

CTG – cardiotocograph

CV – (1) cardiovascular; (2) curriculum vitae

CVA – cerebrovascular accident

CVP – central venous pressure

CVS – (1) cardiovascular system; (2) chorionic villus sampling

CVVH – continuous venous–venous haemofiltration

CVVHD – continuous venous–venous haemodialfiltration

Cx – cervix

CXR – chest X-ray

D

DADL – Domestic Activities of Daily Living

D&C – dilatation and curettage

DC – direct current

DDH – developmental dysplasia of the hip

DIC – disseminated intravascular coagulation

DipEd – Diploma in Education

DipHE – Diploma in Higher Education

DipN – Diploma in Nursing

DipNEd – Diploma in Nursing Education

DKA – diabetic ketoacidosis

DM – diabetes mellitus

DN – district nurse

DNA – (1) deoxyribonucleic acid; (2) did not attend

DOA – dead on arrival

DOB – date of birth

DoH – Department of Health

DPhil – Doctor of Philosophy

DRS – Delusions Rating Scale

DRV – dietary reference value

DSH – deliberate self-harm

DT – delirium tremens

DTPer – diphtheria, tetanus and pertussis vaccine

DU – duodenal ulcer

DVT – deep venous thrombosis

D&V – diarrhoea and vomiting

DXR – deep X-ray radiation

DXT – deep X-ray therapy

E

EAR – estimated average requirement

EBM – expressed breast milk

EBP – evidence-based practice

EBS – emergency bed service

EBV – Epstein–Barr virus

ECF – extracellular fluid

ECG – electrocardiogram

ECI – Experience of Caregiving Inventory

ECMO – extracorporeal membrane oxygenator

ECT – electroconvulsive therapy

EDC – expected date of confinement

EDD – expected date of delivery

EEG – electroencephalogram

EFAs – essential fatty acids

ELISA – enzyme-linked immunosorbent assay

EMD – electromechanical dissociation

EMG – electromyography

EMLA – eutectic mixture of local anaesthetics

EMU – early morning specimen of urine

ENT – ears, nose and throat

EOG – electro-oculogram

ERCP – endoscopic retrograde cholangiopancreatography

ERG – electroretinogram

ERPC – evacuation of retained products of conception

ERV – expiratory reserve volume

ESR – erythrocyte sedimentation rate
ESRD – end-stage renal disease
ESS – Early Signs Scale
ESWL – extracorporeal shock wave lithotripsy
ET – (1) embryo transfer; (2) endotracheal
EUA – examination under anaesthesia

F

F – (1) Fahrenheit (temperature scale); (2) female
FAS – fetal alcohol syndrome
FB – foreign body
FBC – full blood count
FBS – fasting blood sugar
FETC – Further Education Teaching Certificate
FEV – forced expiratory volume
FFP – fresh frozen plasma
FH – (1) family history; (2) fetal heart
FHH – fetal heart heard
FHNH – fetal heart not heard
FMF – fetal movement felt
FPC – Family Planning Clinic
FPCert – Family Planning Certificate
FRC – functional residual capacity

FRCN – Fellow of the Royal College of Nursing
FSH – follicle stimulating hormone
FTND – full-term normal delivery
FVC – forced vital capacity

G

g – gram
GA – general anaesthetic
GC – gonococcus
GCS – Glasgow Coma Scale
GFR – glomerular filtration rate
GGT – γ-glutamyl transferase
GH – growth hormone
GHQ – General Health Questionnaire
GI – gastrointestinal
GIFT – gamete intrafallopian transfer
GIT – gastrointestinal tract
GOR – gastro-oesophageal reflux
GP – general practitioner
GSL – General Sales List (medicines)
GTN – glyceryl trinitrate
GTT – glucose tolerance test
GU – (1) gastric ulcer; (2) genitourinary
GUM – genitourinary medicine
GUS – genitourinary system

GVHD – graft versus host disease

Gyn – gynaecology

H

HAI – hospital-acquired infection

HAV – hepatitis A virus

HAVS – hand–arm vibration syndrome

Hb – haemoglobin

HBIG – hepatitis B immunoglobulin

HBV – hepatitis B virus

HC – head circumference

HCA – healthcare assistant

HCG (hCG) – human chorionic gonadotrophin

HCV – hepatitis C virus

HDL – high-density lipoprotein

HDSU – Hospital Disinfection and Sterilisation Unit

HDU – High Dependency Unit

HDV – hepatitis D virus

HEV – hepatitis E virus

HFEA – Human Fertilisation and Embryology Authority

HHNK – hyperglycaemic hyperosmolar non-ketotic

HI – head injury

Hib vaccine – *Haemophilus influenzae* type B vaccine

HImP – Health Improvement Programme

HIV – human immunodeficiency virus

HNPU – has not passed urine

HoNOS – Health of the Nation Outcome Scale

HPA – Health Protection Agency

HPV – human papilloma virus

HR – heart rate

HRS – Hallucinations Rating Scale

HRT – hormone-replacement therapy

HSV – herpes simplex virus

Ht – height

HUS – haemolytic uraemic syndrome

HV – Health Visitor

HVCert – Health Visitor's Certificate

HVT – Health Visitor Teacher

I

IABP – intra-aortic balloon pump

IADL – Instrumental Activities of Daily Living

IBD – inflammatory bowel disease

IBS – irritable bowel syndrome

IC – inspiratory capacity

ICD – International Classification of Disease

ICE – ice, compress and elevate

ICF – intracellular fluid

ICN – (1) Infection Control Nurse; (2) International Council of Nurses

ICP – intracranial pressure

ICSH – interstitial cell stimulating hormone

ICU – Intensive Care Unit

ID – infectious disease

IDDM – insulin-dependent diabetes mellitus

IE – infective endocarditis

IGT – impaired glucose tolerance

IHD – ischaemic heart disease

IM – (1) infectious mononucleosis; (2) intramuscular

IMV – intermittent mandatory ventilation

INR – (1) Index of Nursing Research; (2) international normalised ratio

IOL – intraocular lens

IOP – intraocular pressure

IPD – intermittent peritoneal dialysis

IPP – intermittent positive pressure

IPPV – intermittent positive pressure ventilation

IQ – intelligence quotient

IRV – inspiratory reserve volume

IS – Insight Scale

IT – information technology

ITU – Intensive Therapy Unit

IU – international unit

IUD – intrauterine (contraceptive) device

IUI – intrauterine insemination

IV – intravenous

IVC – inferior vena cava

IVF – *in vitro* fertilisation

IVI – intravenous infusion

IVU – intravenous urogram

J

JCA – juvenile chronic arthritis

JVP – jugular venous pressure

K

KASI – Knowledge about Schizophrenia Interview

KS – Kaposi's sarcoma

KUB – kidney, ureter and bladder

L

L, l – litre

LA – (1) left atrium; (2) local anaesthetic; (3) local authority

lb – pound (of weight)

LBP – low back pain

LDH – lactate dehydrogenase

LDL – low-density lipoprotein

LDQ – Leeds Dependence Questionnaire

LFTs – liver function tests

LH – luteinising hormone

LIF – left iliac fossa

LMN – lower motor neuron

LMP – last menstrual period

LOC – level of consciousness

LP – lumbar puncture

LRNI – lower reference nutrient intake

LRTI – lower respiratory tract infection

LSCS – lower segment Caesarean section

LTM – long-term memory

LUNSERS – Liverpool University Neuroleptic Side Effect Rating Scale

LV – left ventricle

LVAD – left ventricular assist device

LVF – left ventricular failure

LVH – left ventricular hypertrophy

M

M – male

MA – Master of Arts

MAC – mid-arm circumference

mane – in the morning (of drugs); tomorrow

MAO – monoamine oxidase inhibitor

MBC – maximal breathing capacity

MCA – Medicines Control Agency (now merged with Medical Devices Agency)

MCH – mean cell haemoglobin

MCHC – mean cell haemoglobin concentration

MCL – mid-clavicular line

MCV – mean cell volume

MDA – Medical Devices Agency (now merged with Medicines Control Agency)

MDR-TB – multidrug resistant tuberculosis

ME – myalgic encephalomyelitis

MEd – Master of Education

M/F; M/W/S/D – male/female; married/widowed/single/divorced

MHRA – Medicines and Healthcare products Regulatory Agency (formed from the MCA and MDA)

MI – (1) mitral incompetence or insufficiency; (2) myocardial infarction

mmHg – millimetres of mercury

mmol – millimole

MMR – measles mumps and rubella (as in vaccine)

MMV – mandatory minute volume

MODS – multiple organ dysfunction syndrome

MODY – maturity onset diabetes of the young

MPhil – Master of Philosophy

MRI – magnetic resonance imaging

MRSA – methicillin-resistant S*taphylococcus aureus*

MS – (1) mitral stenosis; (2) multiple sclerosis; (3) musculoskeletal

MSc – Master of Science

MSH – melanocyte-stimulating hormone

MSP – Munchausen syndrome by proxy

MSU – mid-stream urine

MSW – medical social worker

MT – midwifery teacher

MTD – Midwife Teachers' Diploma

MWO – mental welfare officer

N

NAD – no abnormality detected

NAI – non-accidental injury

NAS – no added salt

NBI – no bone injury

NBM – nil (nothing) by mouth

NCVQ – National Council for Vocational Qualifications

ND – normal delivery

NFA – (1) no fixed abode; (2) no further action

NG – nasogastric

NHL – non-Hodgkin's lymphoma

NHS – National Health Service

NICE – National Institute for Clinical Excellence

NICU – Neonatal Intensive Care Unit

NIDDM – non-insulin-dependent diabetes mellitus

NIPPV – non-invasive positive pressure ventilation

NMC – Nursing and Midwifery Council

NMR – nuclear magnetic resonance

nocte – in the evening (of drugs)

NPF – *Nurse Prescribers' Formulary*

NPU – not passed urine

NRDS – neonatal respiratory distress syndrome

NREM – non-rapid eye movement (sleep)

NSAIDs – non-steroidal anti-inflammatory drugs

NSFs – National Service Frameworks

NSP – non-starch polysaccharides

NSU – non-specific urethritis

NT – nurse teacher

N&V – nausea and vomiting

NVQ – National Vocational Qualification

O

OA – osteoarthritis

OBS – organic brain syndrome

OCD – obsessive–compulsive disorder

o.d. – omni die (Latin – sometimes used in prescriptions), daily

OD – overdose

ODP – operating department practitioner

O/E, OE – on examination

OGD – oesophagogastroduo-denoscopy

OHNC – Occupational Health Nursing Certificate

o.m. – omni mane (Latin – sometimes used in prescriptions), in the morning

o.n. – omni nocte (Latin – sometimes used in prescriptions), at night

ONC – Orthopaedic Nurses' Certificate

OND – Ophthalmic Nursing Diploma

OPCS – Office of Population Censuses and Surveys

OPD – Outpatients Department

ORT – oral rehydration therapy

OT – occupational therapist (therapy)

OTC – over the counter (drugs bought without a prescription)

OU – Open University

P

P – pulse

PAC – premature atrial contraction

PADL – Personal Activities of Daily Living

PAFC – pulmonary artery flotation catheter

PALS – paediatric advanced life support

PANSS – Positive and Negative Syndrome Scale

Pap – Papanicolaou smear test

PAT – paroxysmal atrial tachycardia

PAWP – pulmonary artery wedge pressure

PBD – peak bone density

PBM – peak bone mass

p.c. – post cibum (Latin – sometimes used in prescriptions), after food

PCAG – primary closed-angle glaucoma

PCA(S) – patient-controlled analgesia (system)

PCEA – patient-controlled epidural analgesia

PCM – protein–calorie malnutrition

PCP – *Pneumocystis carinii* pneumonia

PCT – Primary Care Trust

PCV – packed cell volume

PCWP – pulmonary capillary wedge pressure

PD – peritoneal dialysis

PDA – patent ductus arteriosus

PDP – personal development plan

PE – pulmonary embolus

PEEP – positive end-expiratory pressure

PEFR – peak expiratory flow rate

PEG – percutaneous endoscopic gastrostomy

PEM – protein–energy malnutrition

PET – (1) positron emission tomography; (2) pre-eclamptic toxaemia

PFI – private finance initiative

PFR – peak flow rate

PGL – persistent generalised lymphadenopathy

pH – hydrogen ion concentration

PHCT – Primary Health Care Team

PhD – Doctor of Philosophy

PHLS – Public Health Laboratory Service

PICC – peripherally inserted central catheter

PICU – Paediatric Intensive Care Unit

PID – (1) pelvic inflammatory disease; (2) prolapsed intervertebral disc

PKU – phenylketonuria

PL – perception of light

PM – postmortem

PMB – postmenopausal bleeding

PMH – past medical history

PMS – premenstrual syndrome

PMT – premenstrual tension

PN – postnatal

PND – paroxysmal nocturnal dyspnoea

POAG – primary open-angle glaucoma

POM – prescription only medicine

PONV – postoperative nausea and vomiting

POP – plaster of Paris

PPD – (1) progressive perceptive deafness; (2) purified protein derivative

PPH – post-partum haemorrhage

PPS – plasma protein solution

PPV – positive pressure ventilation

PR – per rectum

PREP – post-registration education and practice

PRL – prolactin

p.r.n. – pro re nata (Latin – sometimes used in prescriptions), when required

PSA – prostate-specific antigen

PSCT – Pain and Symptom Control Team

PSV – pressure support ventilation

PT – (1) physiotherapist; (2) prothrombin

PTA – prior to admission

PTC – percutaneous transhepatic cholangiography

PTCA – percutaneous transluminal coronary angioplasty

PTH – parathyroid hormone

PTSD – post-traumatic stress disorder

PTT – partial thromboplastin time

PU – passed urine

PUFA – polyunsaturated fatty acid

PUO – pyrexia of unknown origin

PV – per vagina

PVD – peripheral vascular disease

PVS – persistent vegetative state

PVT – paroxysmal ventricular tachycardia

Q

QALY – quality-adjusted life-year

q.d.s. – quater die sumendus (Latin – sometimes used in prescriptions), four times a day

q.i.d. – quater in die (Latin), four times a day

QIDN – Queen's Institute of District Nursing

q.q.h. – quarta quaque hora (Latin), every 4 hours

R

R – respiration

RA – (1) rheumatoid arthritis; (2) right atrium

RAI – Relatives' Assessment Interview

RAISSE – Relatives' Assessment Interview for Schizophrenia in a Secure Environment

RBC – (1) red blood cell; (2) red blood cell count

RBS – random blood sugar

RCC – red cell concentrate

RCM – Royal College of Midwives

RCN – Royal College of Nursing and National Council of Nurses of the UK

RCNT – Registered Clinical Nurse Teacher

RCT – randomised controlled trial

RDA – recommended daily allowance

REM – rapid eye movement (sleep)

RG – remedial gymnast

RGN – Registered General Nurse

Rh – rhesus factor

RHD – rheumatic heart disease

RHV – Registered Health Visitor

RICE – rest, ice, compress, elevation

RIF – right iliac fossa

rINN – recommended international non-proprietary name

RIP – raised intracranial pressure

RM – Registered Midwife

RMN – Registered Mental Nurse

RN – Registered Nurse

RNA – ribonucleic acid

RNI – reference nutrient intake

RNIB – Royal National Institute for the Blind

RNID – Royal National Institute for the Deaf

RNMH – Registered Nurse for the Mentally Handicapped

RNT – Registered Nurse Tutor

RO – reality orientation

ROM – range of movement (exercises)

ROS – removal of sutures

RS – respiratory system

RSCN – Registered Sick Children's Nurse

RSI – repetitive strain injury

RSV – respiratory syncytial virus

RTA – (1) renal tubular acidosis; (2) road traffic accident

RTI – respiratory tract infection

RV – (1) residual volume; (2) right ventricle

RVF – right ventricular failure

S

SAD – seasonal affective disorder

SAH – subarachnoidal haemorrhage

SAI – sexually acquired infection

SANS – Schedule for Assessment of Negative Symptoms

SARS – severe acute respiratory syndrome

SC – subcutaneous

SCBU – Special Care Baby Unit

SCC – (1) spinal cord compression; (2) squamous cell carcinoma

SCD – sequential pneumatic compression device

SCM – State Certified Midwife

SDAT – senile dementia Alzheimer type

SDH – subdural haematoma

SERMs – selective (o)estrogen receptor modulators

SFS – Social Functioning Scale

SG – specific gravity

SGA – small for gestational age

SHHD – Scottish Home and Health Department

SHO – senior house officer

SI Units – Système International d'Unités

SIB – self-injurious behaviour

SIDS – sudden infant death syndrome

SIMV – synchronised intermittent mandatory ventilation

SLE – systemic lupus erythematosus

SLS – social and life skills

SLT – speech and language therapist (therapy)

SMR – (1) standardised mortality rate; (2) submucous resection

SNAP – Schizophrenia Nursing Assessment Protocol

SOB – short of breath

SPECT – single photon emission computed tomography

SPF – sun protection factor

SRN – State Registered Nurse

SSRIs – selective serotonin re-uptake inhibitors

stat. – statim (Latin – sometimes used in prescriptions), immediately

STD – sexually transmitted disease

STI – sexually transmitted infection

STM – short-term memory

STs – sanitary towels

SVC – superior vena cava

SVQs – Scottish Vocational Qualifications

SVT – supraventricular tachycardia

SWD – short-wave diathermy

T

T – temperature

T&A – tonsils and adenoids

TB – tuberculosis

TCA – tricyclic antidepressants

TCI – to come in

t.d.s. – ter die sumendus (Latin – sometimes used in prescriptions), three times a day

TEDs – thromboembolic deterrent (stockings)

TEN – toxic epidermal necrolysis

TENS – transcutaneous electrical nerve stimulation

TIA – transient ischaemic attack

t.i.d. – ter in die (Latin), three times a day

TIPSS – transjugular intrahepatic portasystemic stent shunting

TLC – total lung capacity

TLS – tumour lysis syndrome

TNF – tumour necrosis factor

TNM – tumour, node, metastasis

TOP – termination of pregnancy

TPN – total parenteral nutrition

TPR – temperature, pulse, respiration

TRIC – trachoma inclusion conjunctivitis

TSF – triceps skin-fold thickness

TSH – thyroid-stimulating hormone

TSS – toxic shock syndrome

TT – (1) tetanus toxoid; (2) thrombin clotting time; (3) tuberculin tested

TTA(O) – to take away (out)

TUR – transurethral resection

TURP – transurethral resection of the prostate gland

TURT – transurethral resection of tumour

TV – (1) tidal volume; (2) *Trichomonas vaginalis*

U

U – unit

U&E – urea and electrolytes

UG – urogenital

UGS – urogenital system

UGT – urogenital tract

UKCC – UK Central Council for Nursing, Midwifery and Health Visiting (replaced by Nursing and Midwifery Council)

UMN – upper motor neuron

URTI – upper respiratory tract infection

USS – ultrasound scan

UTI – urinary tract infection

UVA – ultraviolet A

UVB – ultraviolet B

UVL – ultraviolet light

V

VA – visual acuity
VAS – visual analogue scale
VBI – vertebrobasilar insufficiency
VC – vital capacity
VD – venereal disease (outdated term)
VE – vaginal examination
VF – ventricular fibrillation
VFM – value for money
VLDL – very-low-density lipoprotein
VRE – vancomycin-resistant enterococci
VRS – Verbal Rating Scale
VSD – ventricular septal defect
VT – ventricular tachycardia
VUR – vesicoureteric reflux

VV – varicose vein(s)
VZIG – varicella-zoster immunoglobulin
VZV – varicella-zoster virus

W

WBC – (1) white blood cell; (2) white blood cell count
WC – water closet (lavatory)
WHO – World Health Organisation
WPW – Wolff–Parkinson–White syndrome
Wt – weight

Z

ZIFT – zygote intrafallopian transfer
ZN – Ziehl–Neelsen (stain)

Useful addresses and web sources

10

Some useful addresses and web sources are provided in this chapter. They will help you to get up-to-date information about the sort of issues that are important for a satisfying and successful nursing career in the UK. These include: immigration, registration as a nurse in the UK, welfare and employment, and education opportunities. Also included are some sources of information for your patients and their families.

INFORMATION FOR NURSES

Addresses and websites

Commission for Racial Equality
Elliot House
10–12 Allington Street
London SW1E 5EH
http://www.cre.gov.uk

Commonwealth Nurses Federation
c/o International Department
Royal College of Nursing
20 Cavendish Square
London W1M 0AB

Community and District Nursing Association (CDNA)
Westel House
32–38 Uxbridge Road
Ealing
London W5 2BS
http://www.cdna.tvu.ac.uk

Community Practitioners' and Health Visitors' Association
(CPHVA)
40 Bermondsey Street
London SE1 3UD
http://www.amicus-cphva.org
(Affiliated to Amicus)

Department of Health
Richmond House
79 Whitehall
London SW1A 2NS
http://www.dh.gov.uk

Equal Opportunities Commission
Arndale House
Arndale Centre
Manchester M4 5EQ
http://www.eoc.org.uk

GMB
22/24 Worple Road
London SW19 4DD
http://www.gmb.org.uk

Health & Safety Executive
Rose Court
2 Southwark Bridge
London SE1 9HS
http://www.hse.gov.uk

Health Service Commissioner
13th Floor Millbank
Millbank Tower
London SW1P 4QP
http://www.health.ombudsman.org.uk

HM Customs and Excise
Dorset House
Stamford Street
London SE1 9PY
http://www.hmce.gov.uk
(Advice on bringing personal effects and goods into the UK)

Home Office
Immigration and Nationality Enquiry Bureau
Block C
Whitgift Centre
Wellesley Road
Croydon CR9 1AT
http://www.homeoffice.gov.uk
(Immigration and Nationality – information on entry visas and work permits)

Immigration Advisory Service (IAS)
County House
190 Great Dover Street
London SE1 4YB
http://www.iasuk.org
(Independent charity that gives free confidential advice and help with applying for entry clearance to the UK)

International Confederation of Midwives
10 Barley Mow Passage
London W4 4PH

International Council of Nurses (ICN)
3 Place Jean Marteau
1201 Geneva
Switzerland
http://www.icn.ch

Mental Health Nurses' Association (formerly CPNA)
Cals Meyn
Grove Lane
Hinton
Nr Chippenham
Wilts SN14 8HF
(Affiliated to Amicus)

Nurses Welfare Service
Victoria Chambers
16/18 Strutton Ground
London SW1P 2HP

Nursing and Midwifery Council (NMC)
Overseas Registration
23 Portland Place
London W1N 3PZ
http://www.nmc-uk.org
(Provides information about registering as a nurse or midwife in the UK)

Royal College of Midwives
15 Mansfield Street
London W1G 9NH
http://www.rcm.org.uk

Royal College of Nursing of the United Kingdom
20 Cavendish Square
London W1M 0AB
http://www.rcn.org.uk/whyjoin/howtojoin
(Provides general information on how to become registered as a nurse in the UK)

Royal Commonwealth Society
18 Northumberland Avenue
London WC2N 5BJ

Scottish Health Department
St. Andrew's House
Regent Road
Edinburgh EH1 3DE
http://www.scotland.gov.uk

Unison (Head Office)
1 Mabledon Place
London WC1H 9HA
http://www.unison.org.uk

World Health Organisation
Avenue Appia
1211 Geneva 27
Switzerland
http://www.who.org

Web resources

Citizens Advice Bureaux (CAB) – give free advice on many issues. Branches can be found in most large towns and cities: http://www.adviceguide.org.uk

Foreign and Commonwealth Office – gives details about visa requirements for visitors wishing to enter the UK: http://www.fco.gov.uk

International English Language Testing System – useful information about the IELTS test and the centres which run the test, etc.: http://www.ielts.org

Nursing courses – full guide to nursing courses in the UK: http://www.nursingcourses.co.uk

Nursing in the UK – information about immigration procedures: http://www.nursingintheuk.co.uk

NursingNetUK – information about nursing in the UK, job vacancies and courses: http://www.nursingnetuk.com

Nursing Times – information about the weekly journal, nursing issues, and job vacancies on NT Job Alert: http://www.nursingtimes.net

Office of the Immigration Services Commissioner – UK government regulator for immigration services. Information and complaints: http://www.oisc.gov.uk

University of Sheffield School of Nursing and Midwifery – supports international students in a wide variety of academic programmes:
http://www.snm.shef.ac.uk/snm/internat/internat.htm

INFORMATION FOR PATIENTS AND FAMILIES

Addresses and websites

Action for Sick Children
300 Kingston Road
London SW20 8LX
http://www.actionforsickchildren.org

Age Concern (England)
1268 London Road
London SW16 4ER
http://www.ace.org.uk

Alcoholics Anonymous
PO Box 1
Stonebow House
Stonebow
York YO1 2NJ
http://www.alcoholics-anonymous.org.uk

Alzheimer's Society
Gordon House
10 Greencoat Place
London SW1P 1PH
http://www.alzheimers.org.uk

Arthritis Care
18 Stephenson Way
London NW1 2HD
http://www.arthritiscare.org.uk

Association of Carers
20–25 Glasshouse Yard
London EC1A 4JS

Breast Cancer Care
Kiln House
210 New King's Road
London SW6 4NZ
http://www.breastcancercare.org.uk

British Association for Cancer United Patients BACUP
3 Bath Place
Rivington Street
London EC2 3JR
http://www.cancerbacup.org.uk

British Colostomy Association
15 Station Road
Reading RG1 1LG
http://www.bcass.org.uk

British Deaf Association
1–3 Worship Street
London EC2A 2AB
http://www.bda.org.uk

British Epilepsy Association
New Anstey House
Gate Way Drive
Leeds LS3 1BE
http://www.epilepsy.org.uk

British Heart Foundation
14 Fitzhardinge Street
London W1H 4DH
http://www.bhf.org.uk

British Pregnancy Advisory Service
Austy Manor
Wootton Wawen
Solihull
West Midlands B95 6BX
http://www.bpas.org.uk

British Red Cross
9 Grosvenor Crescent
London SW1X 7EJ
http://www.redcross.org.uk

Capability *(formerly Spastics Society)*
12 Park Crescent
London W1N 4EQ

Diabetes UK
10 Queen Anne Street
London W1M 0BD
http://www.diabetes.org.uk

Disabled Living Foundation
380–384 Harrow Road
London W9 2HU
http://www.dlf.org.uk

Ileostomy & Internal Pouch Support Group
Amblehurst House
PO Box 23
Mansfield NG18 4TT

Leukaemia Society
14 Kingfisher Court
Venny Bridge
Pinhoe
Exeter EX4 8JN

Macmillan Cancer Relief
89 Albert Embankment
London SE1 7UQ
http://www.macmillan.org.uk

MIND – National Association for Mental Health
Granta House
15–19 Broadway
London E15 4BQ
http://www.mind.org.uk

Multiple Sclerosis Society
National Centre
372 Edgware Road
London NW2 6ND
http://www.mssociety.org.uk

National Aids Trust
New City Cloisters
196 Old Street
London EC1V 9FR
http://www.nat.org.uk

National Asthma Campaign
Providence House
Providence Place
London N1 0NT
http://www.asthma.org.uk

National Society for the Prevention of Cruelty to Children
  (NSPCC)
42 Curtain Road
London EC2A 3NH
http://www.nspcc.org.uk

Royal National Institute of the Blind (RNIB)
105 Judd Street
London WC1H 9NE
http://www.rnib.org.uk

Royal National Institute for the Deaf (RNID)
19–23 Featherstone Street
London EC1Y 8SL
http://www.rnid.org.uk

St. Andrews Ambulance Association
St. Andrew's House
48 Milton Street
Glasgow G4 0HR
http://www.firstaid.org.uk

St. John Ambulance Association & Brigade
1 Grosvenor Crescent
London SW1X 7EF
http://www.sja.org.uk

Sickle Cell Society
54 Station Road
Harlesden
London NW10 4UA
http://www.sicklecellsociety.org

Stillbirth & Neonatal Death Society (SANDS)
28 Portland Place
London W1N 4DE

Stroke Association
123–127 Whitecross Street
London EC1Y 8JJ
http://www.stroke.org.uk

Terrence Higgins Trust
52–54 Grays Inn Road
London WC1X 8JU
http://www.tht.org.uk

Units of measurement 11

UNITS OF MEASUREMENT: INTERNATIONAL SYSTEM OF UNITS (SI), THE METRIC SYSTEM AND CONVERSIONS

In the UK we use the International System of Units (SI) or Système International d'Unités measurement system for scientific, medical and technical purposes. The SI units have replaced those of the Imperial System. For example, the kilogram is used for weight (or mass) instead of the pound, and the metre for length instead of yards, feet and inches. However, in everyday life you will still see a mix of units used in shops and hear people talk about pounds, and feet and inches. For example, they will ask for a pound of apples and describe someone being 5 foot 3 inches in height and 10 stone in weight.

The SI comprises seven base units, with several derived units. Each unit has its own symbol and is expressed as a decimal multiple or submultiple of the base unit by using the appropriate prefix (e.g. a millimetre is one-thousandth of a metre).

Base units

Quantity	Base unit and symbol
Length	metre (m)
Mass	kilogram (kg)
Time	second (s)
Amount of substance	mole (mol)
Electric current	ampere (A)
Thermodynamic temperature	kelvin (°K)
Luminous intensity	candela (cd)

Derived units

Derived units for measuring different quantities are reached by multiplying or dividing two or more of the seven base units.

Quantity	Derived unit and symbol
Work, energy, quantity of heat	joule (J)
Pressure	pascal (Pa)
Force	newton (N)
Frequency	hertz (Hz)
Power	watt (W)
Electrical potential, electromotive force, potential difference	volt (v)
Absorbed dose of radiation	gray (Gy)
Radioactivity	becquerel (Bq)
Dose equivalent	sievert (Sv)

Factor, decimal multiples and submultiples of SI units

Multiplication factor	Prefix	Symbol
10^{12}	tera	T
10^9	giga	G
10^6	mega	M
10^3	kilo	k
10^2	hecto	h
10^1	deca	da
10^{-1}	deci	d
10^{-2}	centi	c
10^{-3}	milli	m
10^{-6}	micro	μ
10^{-9}	nano	n
10^{-12}	pico	p
10^{-15}	femto	f
10^{-18}	atto	A

Rules for using units and writing large numbers and decimals

— The symbol for a unit is unaltered in the plural and should not be followed by a full stop/point except at the end of a sentence: i.e. 2 cm, not 2 cm. or 2 cms.

— Large numbers are written in three-digit groups (working from right to left) with spaces not commas (in some countries the comma is used to indicate a decimal point): e.g. forty thousand is written as 40 000, four-hundred thousand is written as 400 000.

— Numbers with four numbers are written without the space: e.g. six thousand is written as 6000.

— The decimal sign between numbers is indicated by a full stop/point placed near the line: e.g. 40.75. If the numerical value of the decimal is less than 1, a zero should appear before the decimal sign: i.e. 0.125, not .125.

— Decimals with more than four numbers are also written in three-digit groups, but this time working from left to right: e.g. 0.000 25.

— 'Squared' and 'cubed' are expressed as numerical powers and not by abbreviation: e.g. square centimetre is cm^2, not sq. cm.

Commonly used measurements requiring further explanation

— *Volume:* volume is calculated by multiplying length, width and depth. Using the SI unit for length, the metre (m), means ending up with a cubic metre (m^3), which is a huge volume and it is not appropriate for most uses. In clinical practice the litre (L or l) is used. A litre is based on the volume of a cube measuring 10 cm × 10 cm × 10 cm. Smaller units still, e.g. millilitre (mL) or one-thousandth of a litre, are commonly used in clinical practice.

— *Pressure:* the SI unit of pressure is the pascal (Pa), and the kilopascal (kPa) replaces the old non-SI unit of millimetres of mercury pressure (mmHg) for blood pressure and blood gases. However, mmHg are still widely used for measuring blood pressure. Other anomalies include: cerebrospinal fluid, which is measured in millimetres of water (mmH_2O); and central venous pressure, which is measured in centimetres of water (cmH_2O).

— *Temperature:* although the SI base unit for temperature is the kelvin, by international convention temperature is measured in degrees Celsius (°C).

— *Energy:* the energy of food or individual requirements for energy are measured in kilojoules (kJ); the SI unit is the joule (J). In practice, many people still use the kilocalorie (kcal), a non-SI unit, for these uses. 1 calorie = 4.2 J; 1 kilocalorie (large Calorie) = 4.2 kJ.

— *Time:* the SI base unit for time is the second (s), but it is acceptable to use minute (min), hour (h) or day (d). In clinical practice it is preferable to use 'per 24 hours' for the excretion of substances in urine and faeces: i.e. g/24 h.

— *Amount of substance:* the SI base unit for amount of substance is the mole (mol). The concentration of many substances is expressed in moles per litre (mol/L) or millimoles per litre (mmol/L), which replaces milliequivalents per litre (mEq/L). Some exceptions exist and include: haemoglobin and plasma proteins, which are given in grams per litre (g/L); and enzyme activity, which is given in International Units (IU, U or iu).

MEASUREMENTS, EQUIVALENTS AND CONVERSIONS (SI OR METRIC AND IMPERIAL)

Volume

1 litre (L) = 1000 millilitres (mL)

1 millilitre (mL) = 1000 microlitres (µL)

Note: The millilitre (mL) and the cubic centimetre (cm^3) are usually treated as being equivalent.

Conversions

> 1 litre (L) = 1.76 pints (pt)
>
> 568.25 millilitres (mL) = 1 pint (pt)
>
> 28.4 millilitres (mL) = 1 fluid ounce (fl oz)

Length

> 1 kilometre (km) = 1000 metres (m)
>
> 1 metre (m) = 100 centimetres (cm) or 1000 millimetres (mm)
>
> 1 centimetre (cm) = 10 millimetres (mm)
>
> 1 millimetre (mm) = 1000 micrometres (μm)
>
> 1 micrometre (μm) = 1000 nanometres (nm)

Conversions

> 1 metre (m) = 39.370 inches (in)
>
> 1 centimetre (cm) = 0.3937 inches (in)
>
> 30.48 centimetres (cm) = 1 foot (ft)
>
> 2.54 centimetres (cm) = 1 inch (in)

Weight or mass

> 1 kilogram (kg) = 1000 grams (g)
>
> 1 gram (g) = 1000 milligrams (mg)
>
> 1 milligram (mg) = 1000 micrograms (μg)
>
> 1 microgram (μg) = 1000 nanograms (ng)

Note: To avoid any confusion with milligram (mg) the word microgram (μg) should be written in full on prescriptions.

Conversions

    1 kilogram (kg) = 2.204 pounds (lb)

    1 gram (g) = 0.0353 ounce (oz)

    453.59 grams (g) = 1 pound (lb)

    28.34 grams (g) = 1 ounce (oz)

Temperature conversions

To convert Celsius to Fahrenheit, multiply by 9, divide by 5, and add 32 to the result. For example, to convert 36°C to Fahrenheit:

    $36 \times 9 = 324 \div 5 = 64.8 + 32 = 96.8°F$

therefore 36°C = 96.8°F.

To convert Fahrenheit to Celsius, subtract 32, multiply by 5, and divide by 9. For example, to convert 104°F to Celsius:

    $104 - 32 = 72 \times 5 = 360 \div 9 = 40°C$

therefore 104°F = 40°C.

Temperature comparison

°Celsius	°Fahrenheit
100	212
95	203
90	194
85	185
80	176
75	167
70	158
65	149
60	140
55	131
50	122
45	113

°Celsius	°Fahrenheit
44	112.2
43	109.4
42	107.6
41	105.8
40	104
39.5	103.1
39	102.2
38.5	101.3
38	100.4
37.5	99.5
37	98.6
36.5	97.7
36	96.8
35.5	95.9
35	95
34	93.2
33	91.4
32	89.6
31	87.8
30	86
25	77
20	68
15	59
10	50
5	41
0	32
−5	23
−10	14

Note:

Boiling point = 100°C = 212°F
Freezing point = 0°C = 32°F

FURTHER READING

Gatford JD, Phillips N 2002 Nursing calculations, 6th edn. Churchill Livingstone, Edinburgh.

General further reading suggestions

Brooker C (ed) 2002 Churchill Livingstone's dictionary of nursing, 18th edn. Churchill Livingstone, Edinburgh.

Brooker C, Nicol M (eds) 2003 Nursing adults: the practice of caring. Mosby, Edinburgh.

Ellis RB, Gates B, Kenworthy N 2003 Interpersonal communication in nursing. Churchill Livingstone, Edinburgh.

Gunn C 2001 Using maths in health sciences. Churchill Livingstone, Edinburgh.

Hoban V 2003 How to ... communicate better with your colleagues. Nursing Times 99:64–65.

Hutton A 2002 An introduction to medical terminology for health care. A self-teaching package, 3rd edn. Churchill Livingstone, Edinburgh.

MacConnachie AM, Hay J, Harris J, Nimmo S 2002 Drugs in nursing practice. An A–Z guide, 6th edn. Churchill Livingstone, Edinburgh.

Nicol M, Bavin C, Bedford-Turner S, et al 2004 Essential nursing skills, 2nd edn. Mosby, Edinburgh.

Richards A, Edwards S 2003 A nurse's survival guide to the ward. Churchill Livingstone, Edinburgh.

Royal College of Nursing (RCN) 2003 Here to stay. International nurses in the UK. Available:
www.rcn.org.uk/professional/publications/heretostay-irns.pdf

Wallace M 2002 Churchill Livingstone's A–Z guide to professional healthcare. Churchill Livingstone, Edinburgh.

Index

'Don't let fear hold you back.
You're **braver** than you think!'

Join Kitty for an **enchanting**
adventure by the light of the **moon**.

Kitty can **talk to animals** and
has **feline superpowers**.

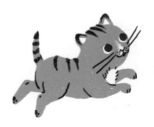

Meet Kitty & her Cat Crew

Kitty

Kitty has special powers but is she ready to be a superhero just like her mum?

Luckily Kitty's Cat Crew have faith in her and show Kitty the hero that lies within!

Pumpkin

A stray ginger kitten who is utterly devoted to Kitty.

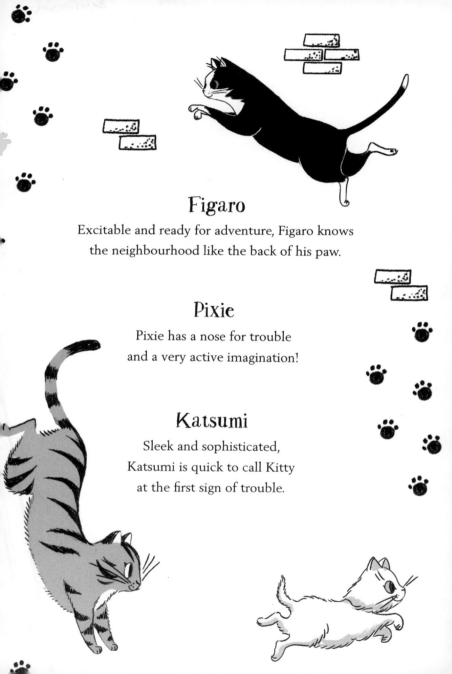

Figaro

Excitable and ready for adventure, Figaro knows
the neighbourhood like the back of his paw.

Pixie

Pixie has a nose for trouble
and a very active imagination!

Katsumi

Sleek and sophisticated,
Katsumi is quick to call Kitty
at the first sign of trouble.

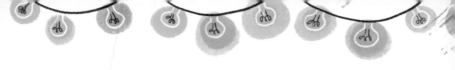

For my mum and dad - P.H.

For Lizzie's little future reader! - J.L.

OXFORD
UNIVERSITY PRESS

Great Clarendon Street, Oxford OX2 6DP

Oxford University Press is a department of the University of Oxford.
It furthers the University's objective of excellence in research, scholarship, and
education by publishing worldwide. Oxford is a registered trade mark of Oxford
University Press in the UK and in certain other countries

Text copyright © Paula Harrison 2021
Illustrations copyright © Jenny Løvlie 2021

The moral rights of the author/illustrator have been asserted
Database right Oxford University Press (maker)

First published 2021

All rights reserved. No part of this publication may be reproduced,
stored in a retrieval system, or transmitted, in any form or by any means,
without the prior permission in writing of Oxford University Press,
or as expressly permitted by law, or under terms agreed with the appropriate
reprographics rights organization. Enquiries concerning reproduction outside
the scope of the above should be sent to the Rights Department, Oxford
University Press, at the address above

You must not circulate this book in any other binding or cover
and you must impose this same condition on any acquirer

British Library Cataloguing in Publication Data

Data available

ISBN: 978-0-19-277170-4

1 3 5 7 9 10 8 6 4 2

Printed in China

Paper used in the production of this book is a natural,
recyclable product made from wood grown in sustainable forests.
The manufacturing process conforms to the environmental
regulations of the country of origin.

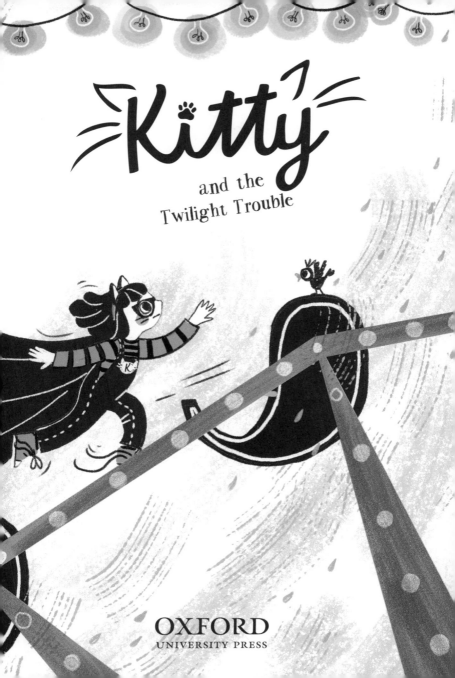

Kitty

and the
Twilight Trouble

OXFORD
UNIVERSITY PRESS

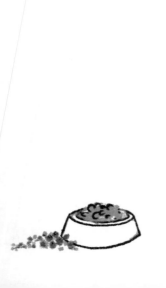

Chapter 1

Kitty bounded across the
school playground at home time.
'Guess what?' She grinned at Dad
and Max, her little brother. 'There's a
funfair setting up on Taylor's Green.'
'Really? That sounds fun!' Dad

1

said, smiling.

'They open tomorrow!' Kitty said breathlessly. 'And there will be rides and toffee apples and everything! The whole class was talking about it today.'

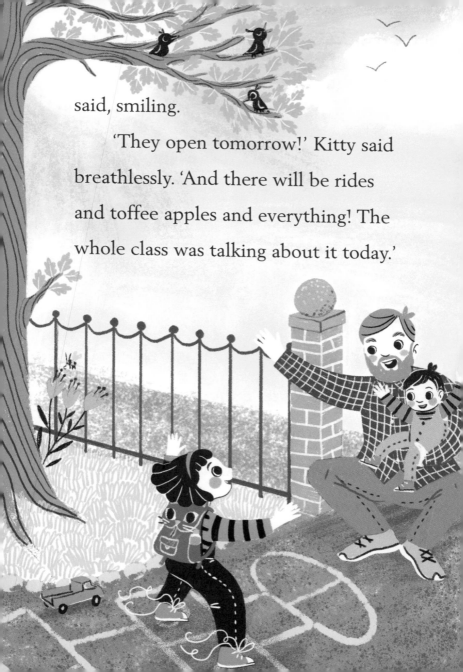

Max's eyes went big and round. 'Ooh, toffee apples!'

Kitty clasped her hands together. 'Can we go? Please?'

'Maybe at the weekend,' Dad replied, steering them towards the school gate. 'Let's see what your mum says.'

Kitty skipped ahead with thoughts of candy floss and rides on the Big Wheel going round in her head. She rushed through the gate into the park. Birds were singing in the treetops and

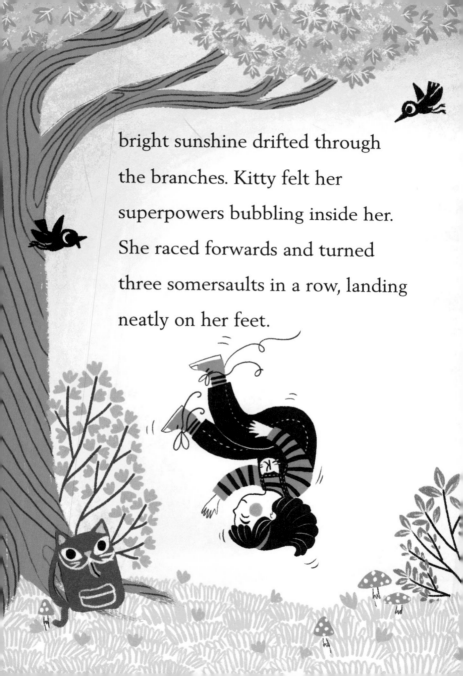

bright sunshine drifted through
the branches. Kitty felt her
superpowers bubbling inside her.
She raced forwards and turned
three somersaults in a row, landing
neatly on her feet.

Kitty had a special secret. She had cat-like superpowers and that was why she could jump and somersault so easily. With her super-powered senses, she could see in the dark and hear sounds from miles away. Her favourite part of being a superhero in training was talking to animals. She loved going on adventures in the moonlight with her cat crew, skipping over the rooftops after dark.

Kitty leapt up to swing off a tree branch. Her dad and Max were quite a way behind and she knew she should wait for them. Suddenly, she glimpsed a furry white cat peeping out from behind a tree trunk. 'Come out, Pixie! I know you're hiding over there.' She grinned. Pixie was one of her cat crew. The little white cat was always full of mischief and loved to play tricks on everyone.

'MIAOW! Got you, Kitty.' Pixie jumped out and pounced on Kitty's foot.

'Hello, Pixie!' Kitty said, laughing.

'What are you doing here?'

'I came to tell you my exciting news!' Pixie's green eyes sparkled. 'I've made a new friend—a cat called Hazel—and she's amazing!'

Kitty smiled. 'I don't think I've met any cats called Hazel.'

'She showed me how to do lots of cool tricks. Just watch this!'

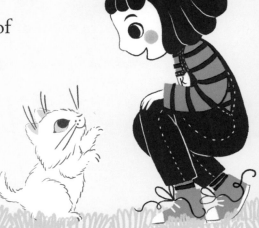
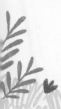

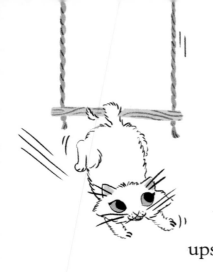

Pixie dashed over to
the play equipment
and leapt on to
the swings, hanging
upside down by her tail.
Then she balanced by the tips of her
paws on the see-saw.

'Brilliant!' said Kitty admiringly.

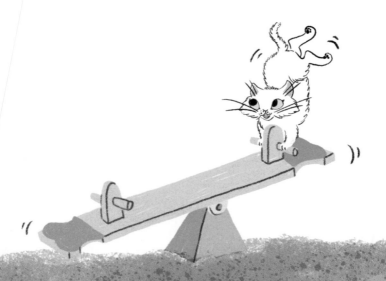

Pixie leapt back down. 'I told her that you're a superhero and I talked about the adventures we've had. She said she'd like to meet you. Can I bring her round tonight?'

'Of course you can!' said Kitty. 'I'd love to meet your friend.'

'Thanks, Kitty! See you soon.' Pixie leapt away through the trees.

Kitty waited for Pixie on her window seat at bedtime. Her best friend, a ginger kitten called Pumpkin, sat snuggled up beside her. Kitty had met Pumpkin on her very first adventure as a superhero in training. Now he lived with her and slept on Kitty's bed every night.

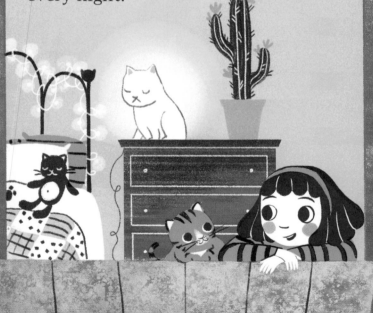

The sky darkened and a bright full moon rose above the flats and houses. Cars with dazzling headlights zoomed along the street below. Kitty peered out of the window, expecting to see Pixie springing jauntily around the chimney pots.

'Are you sure Pixie said she'd come tonight?' Pumpkin asked with a yawn.

'She definitely said tonight.' Kitty frowned a little. 'I wonder if she's changed her mind.'

'I think we should just go to bed.'

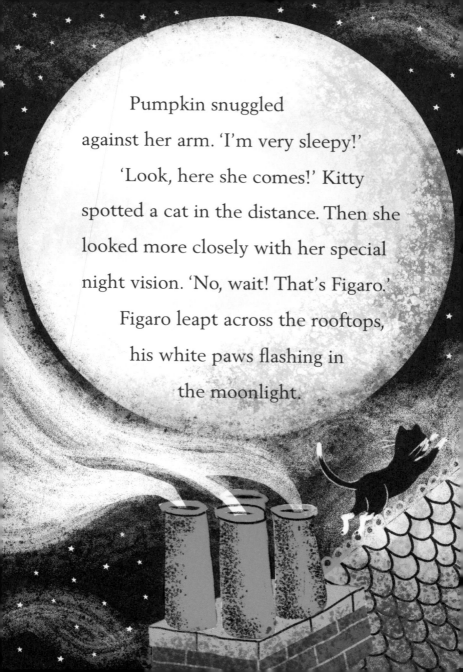

Pumpkin snuggled
against her arm. 'I'm very sleepy!'
'Look, here she comes!' Kitty
spotted a cat in the distance. Then she
looked more closely with her special
night vision. 'No, wait! That's Figaro.'
Figaro leapt across the rooftops,
his white paws flashing in
the moonlight.

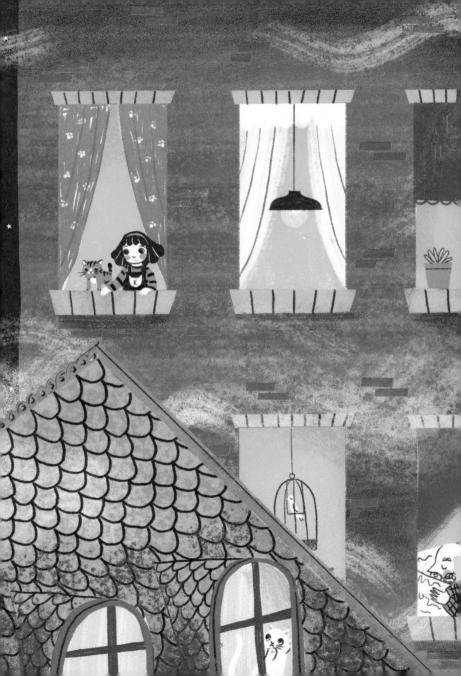

He jumped down to Kitty's windowsill and smoothed his dark whiskers. 'Good evening, Kitty. I'm afraid I bring bad news. I thought it would be best if you heard it straight from me.'

'What's happened?' said Kitty in alarm. 'Does someone need my help?'

Figaro groomed his sleek black fur before replying. 'No, it's about Pixie. She told me she was supposed to come and see you this evening, but she's gone off with another cat instead.'

'Oh! That must be Hazel—her new

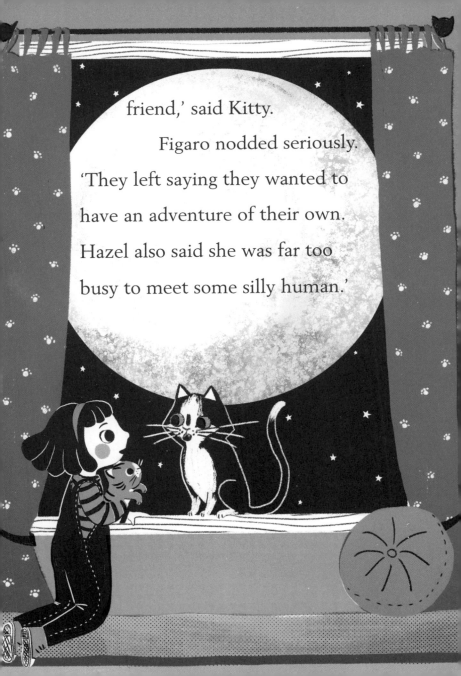

friend,' said Kitty.

Figaro nodded seriously. 'They left saying they wanted to have an adventure of their own. Hazel also said she was far too busy to meet some silly human.'

'That's not very nice!' said
Pumpkin indignantly.

Kitty's heart sank. She'd been
looking forward to meeting Pixie's
new friend. 'Maybe she didn't really
mean it.'

'But there's even MORE!' Figaro's
eyes flashed and he paused, checking
he'd got their attention.

'Hazel said that SHE was
a Cat Superhero with all
kinds of special powers
and that's why they're

having their own adventure. She told me she had important superhero work to do!'

Kitty looked at Figaro in surprise. She hadn't heard of a cat having superpowers before. 'That's amazing! I wonder where they've gone.'

'They didn't tell me.' Figaro sat back and rubbed his ear with one paw. 'I don't like that Hazel though. We used to be a team before she came along.'

'She might be really nice when you get to know her,' Kitty managed to say.

Figaro sniffed and began preening his sleek black-and-white tail.

Kitty gazed out into the darkness. A sprinkling of stars sparkled in the velvet-black sky but thick clouds had hidden the moon.

Kitty didn't want to say bad things about a cat she hadn't even met, but in her heart she agreed with Figaro. She loved her cat crew. They had been on so many great adventures together. She hoped this new cat, Hazel, wasn't going to come along and spoil it all.

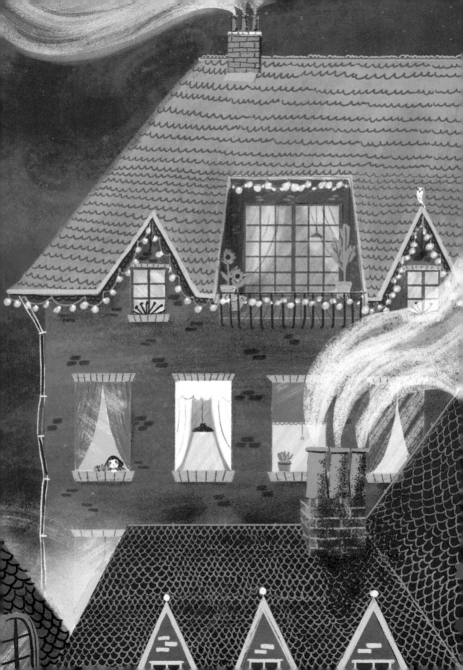

Chapter 2

The moon smiled down on the city like a wise old face the following evening. Kitty waited at her bedroom window again, listening to every tiny sound with her super powered hearing. Cars roared up and down the street,

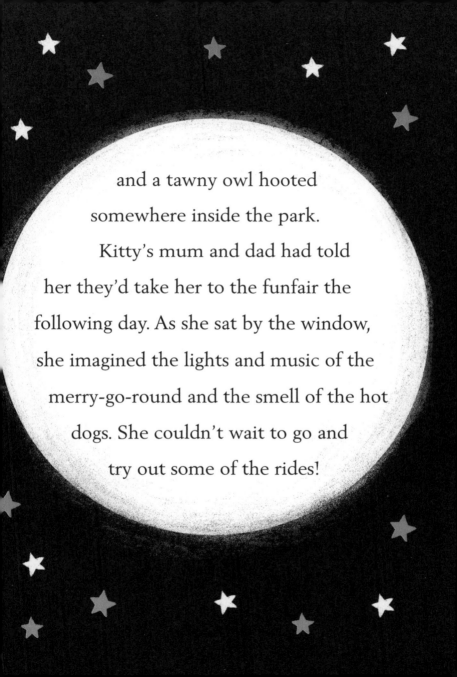

and a tawny owl hooted
somewhere inside the park.

Kitty's mum and dad had told
her they'd take her to the funfair the
following day. As she sat by the window,
she imagined the lights and music of the
merry-go-round and the smell of the hot
dogs. She couldn't wait to go and
try out some of the rides!

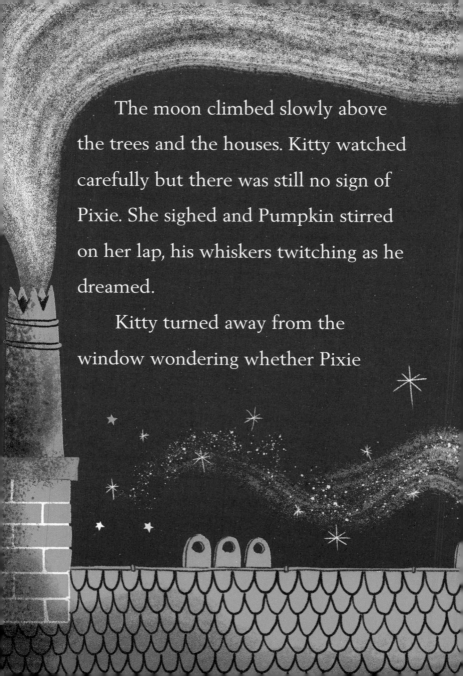

The moon climbed slowly above the trees and the houses. Kitty watched carefully but there was still no sign of Pixie. She sighed and Pumpkin stirred on her lap, his whiskers twitching as he dreamed.

Kitty turned away from the window wondering whether Pixie

didn't want to visit her any more. She was about to lift Pumpkin into her arms and draw the curtain, when she spotted two cats skipping over a distant rooftop. One of them was Pixie with her fluffy white coat gleaming in the moonlight. The other was a brown-and-white tabby with a long sleek tail.

Kitty carefully laid the sleeping Pumpkin on her bed. Then she climbed out of her window and sprang lightly on to the roof. The stars winked in the darkness and a gentle breeze swirled around her. 'Pixie!' she called. 'I'm over here.'

Pixie and her friend carried on playing. They were leaping over a chimney pot and giggling.

Kitty hurried across the rooftops towards them. The other cat must be Hazel, she thought. 'Pixie,' she called.

'I waited for you last night.'

The tabby cat whispered something in Pixie's ear and laughed.

Pixie turned round and skipped over to Kitty. 'Hi Kitty, this is Hazel.' She waved her paw towards the tabby cat.

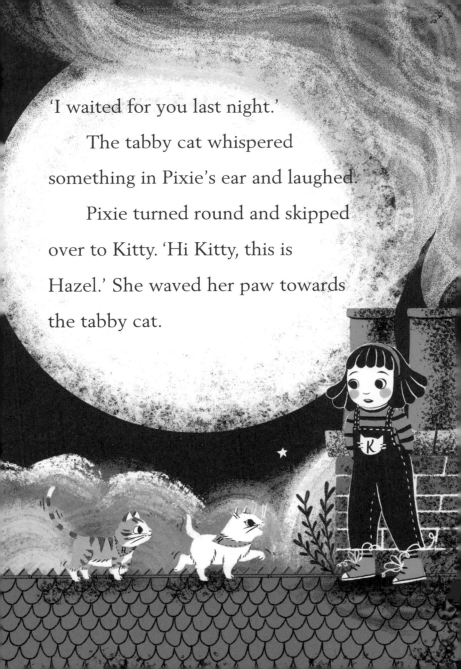

'Hello, Hazel.' Kitty smiled at the tabby, who looked back warily. She noticed that the cats had matching red neckerchiefs tied around their throats. Each one had the letter 'H' sewn on to it.

'Sorry I didn't come to see you yesterday,' said Pixie. 'We were really busy having an adventure.'

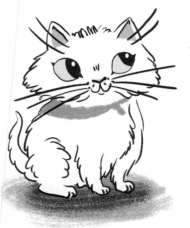

'That sounds like fun!' replied Kitty. 'Wow, I love your matching scarfs.

They look so pretty.'

'Oh, thanks!' Pixie flicked her tail proudly. 'We're wearing them because . . .'

'Shh, don't tell the human!' Hazel gave Pixie a nudge. Then she leapt away across the rooftops. 'Come on, Pixie. I know a great place we can explore.'

Kitty flushed. She was trying to be nice but Hazel didn't seem very interested in being friends.

Pixie hadn't noticed Hazel's rudeness. The little white cat sprang after her new friend, calling back, 'got

27

to go, Kitty! See you tomorrow maybe.'

Kitty watched them dash away over the rooftops. Then she walked slowly back home and climbed through her bedroom window.

'What happened? Is someone in trouble?' Pumpkin asked sleepily.

'Everything's fine, don't worry.' Kitty snuggled down in bed and turned out the light.

Pumpkin went back to sleep but Kitty gazed at the moon peeping through the curtains. Why had Hazel

been so rude when she was only trying
to be friends? Kitty tried to remember
whether she'd said something wrong,
but she didn't think she had.

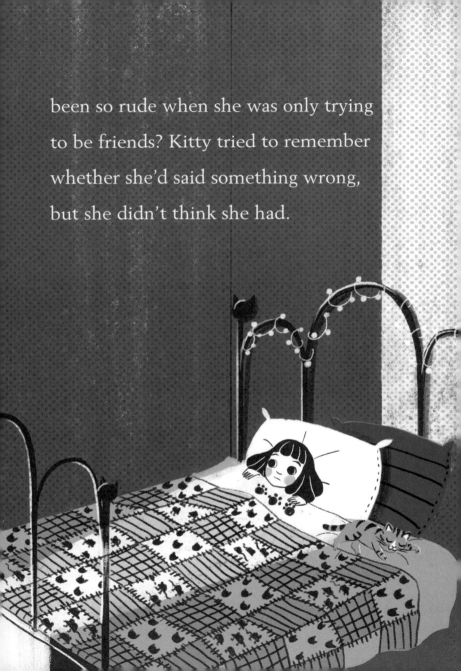

Kitty turned over in bed. She wished Pixie had stopped to talk rather than running off for an adventure. After all, they had been friends long before Hazel came along.

Kitty's mum and dad took Kitty and Max to the funfair after dinner the following day. They walked towards Taylor's Green as the sun set and streaks of orange hung in the sky like bright streamers.

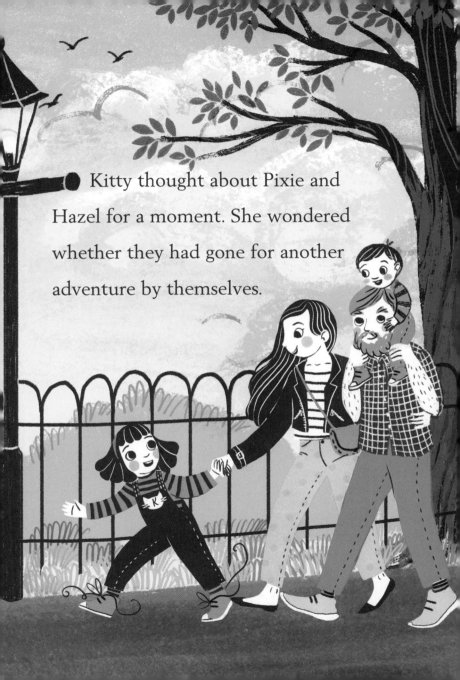

Kitty thought about Pixie and Hazel for a moment. She wondered whether they had gone for another adventure by themselves.

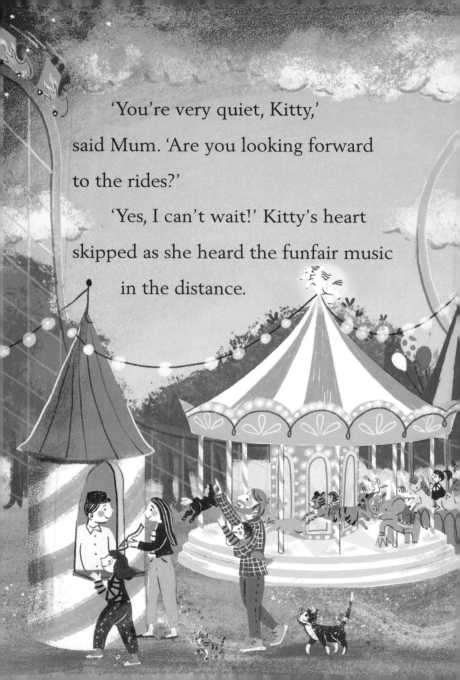

'You're very quiet, Kitty,'
said Mum. 'Are you looking forward
to the rides?'

'Yes, I can't wait!' Kitty's heart
skipped as she heard the funfair music
in the distance.

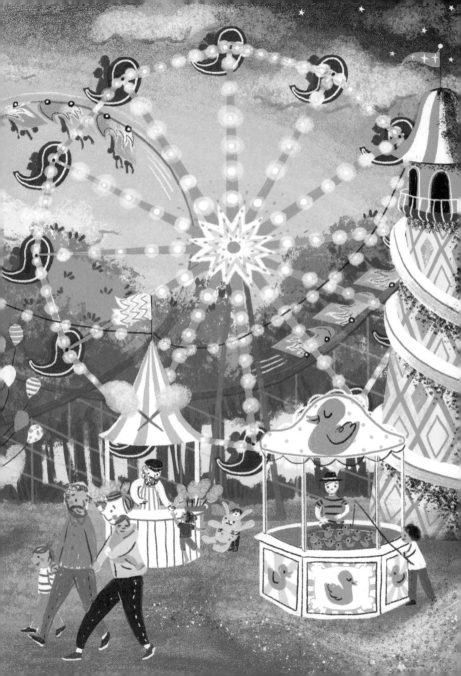

People crowded into the narrow street leading to Taylor's Green and Kitty spotted the Big Wheel with its flashing rainbow lights. The music grew louder and the smell of popcorn and candy floss drifted through the evening air.

Pumpkin and Figaro had decided to come and see what the fair was all about.

Pumpkin gazed around with wide eyes. 'It's very noisy, isn't it?' he said, a little doubtfully.

'Yes, but there is so much to do!'
Figaro leapt on to the Hook-a-Duck
stall and swiped playfully at the plastic
ducks with his paw.

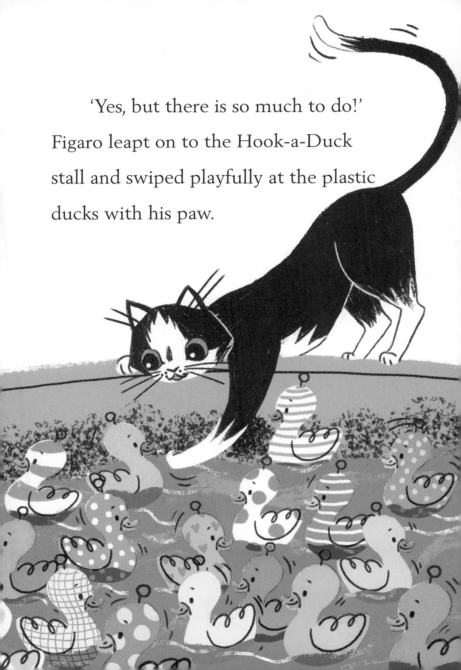

After a moment,
Pumpkin leapt up beside
him and the two cats swiped
at the toy ducks together. Kitty watched
them wistfully. It looked like a fun
game for a cat.

Max asked Kitty to take him
on the Alligator Bounce ride. When
she returned, she found Figaro and
Pumpkin by the toffee apple stall.
Figaro was frowning deeply.

'What's wrong?' asked Kitty.

'It's that Hazel again!' snapped

Figaro. 'She and Pixie are rushing around looking for someone to rescue. It's as if Pixie has forgotten that she was part of *our* cat crew first!'

'Oh!' Kitty sighed. Maybe Pixie thought Hazel was a better superhero than she was.

'I honestly don't know why she's hanging around with Hazel,' Figaro went on. 'We had *millions* of adventures together before that tabby cat came along.'

Kitty took a deep breath. 'But it's nice that they want to help! If you've got superpowers then you should use them to make the world a better place.'

Pumpkin rubbed against her legs. 'There aren't any superheroes as good as you though.'

'Thanks, Pumpkin!' Kitty stroked the kitten's head.

Figaro made a cross harrumphing noise before heading off to the fish and chip stand.

Kitty sighed. Thinking about Pixie and Hazel was starting to make her head ache. 'Come on!' she said to Pumpkin. 'There's a coconut shy over here. Shall I have a go? Maybe I can win a prize.' She handed the stall-holder some coins and he gave her three balls.

While she waited for her turn,
Kitty noticed Pixie and Hazel climbing
up the side of the candy floss stall.
They jumped around, chasing each
other's tails, their matching red scarves
flapping.

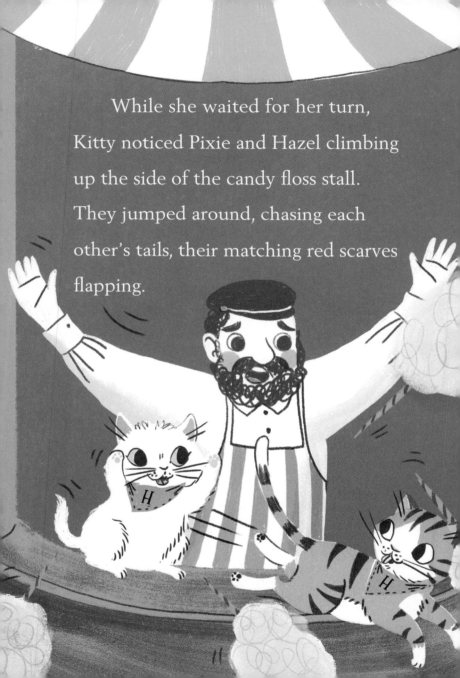

Pixie hung upside down from the stall and swiped some candy floss from a small boy. She stuck her paw in her mouth and licked off the sugary pink mixture.

The little boy noticed his food was gone and began to cry. Hazel giggled.

Kitty frowned. That wasn't superhero behaviour at all.

'Kitty, it's your turn!' said Pumpkin, and Kitty turned back to the coconut shy.

She knocked down the coconuts

one by one and chose a rainbow-coloured bouncy ball as her prize. Her mum and dad came along with Max and they all took turns at knocking the coconuts down. By the time Kitty looked back at the candy floss stall, Pixie and Hazel had disappeared.

'Kitty, I need your help!' Figaro came rushing back, his whiskers twitching in panic. 'There's a whole nest of baby birds in terrible danger. Hurry!'

Kitty and Pumpkin followed Figaro through the crowd. Figaro stopped beside the rollercoaster and clutched his cheek. 'Oh dear, this is terrible! I can't look!'

The rollercoaster went past in a whirl of speed and noise, and the riders shouted out in excitement. Kitty followed Figaro's gaze. An old oak tree stood beside the rollercoaster, with one branch stretching out towards the ride.

Kitty spotted the birds' nest straightaway. It was perched in the

crook of a branch beside the
rollercoaster and every time the
ride zoomed past it juddered a
little closer to the edge. Three
little feathery heads peeped
over the side of the nest. The
birds' eyes were wide with fright
and their tiny wings flapped
helplessly.

Pumpkin gasped. 'The poor

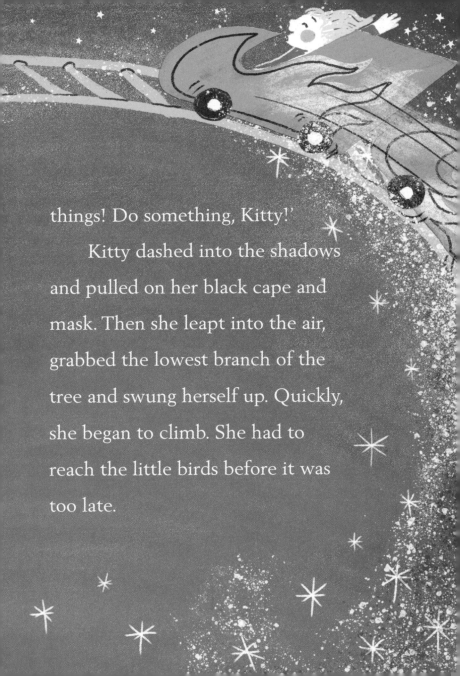

things! Do something, Kitty!'

Kitty dashed into the shadows and pulled on her black cape and mask. Then she leapt into the air, grabbed the lowest branch of the tree and swung herself up. Quickly, she began to climb. She had to reach the little birds before it was too late.

Chapter 3

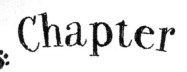

The moonlight poured down and Kitty felt her superpowers tingling inside her. She climbed swiftly, swinging from one branch to the next, hidden in the shadows. Then she shinned up the tree trunk, digging her trainers into the

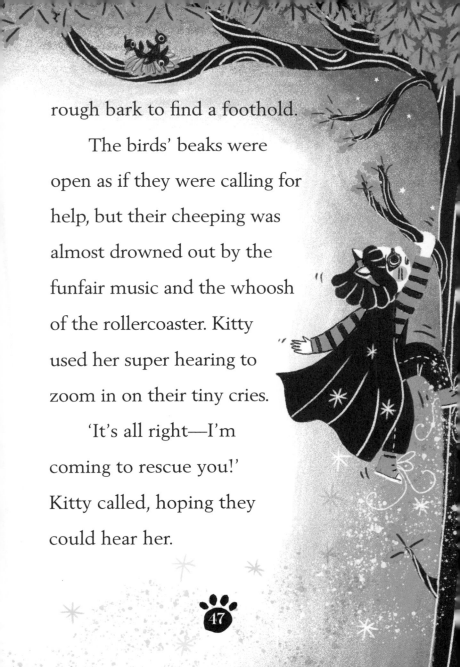

rough bark to find a foothold.

The birds' beaks were
open as if they were calling for
help, but their cheeping was
almost drowned out by the
funfair music and the whoosh
of the rollercoaster. Kitty
used her super hearing to
zoom in on their tiny cries.

'It's all right—I'm
coming to rescue you!'
Kitty called, hoping they
could hear her.

The ride zoomed past, making the tree shake furiously. The flashing lights dazzled Kitty and the screeching machinery made her head ache. But she clung on, holding tight to the branch with her fingertips.

The birds' nest wobbled dangerously as the rollercoaster passed by. Kitty watched in horror as the nest tipped sideways and a tiny feathery shape dangled over the edge. She climbed faster, her heart racing. She had to reach the nest before the ride came

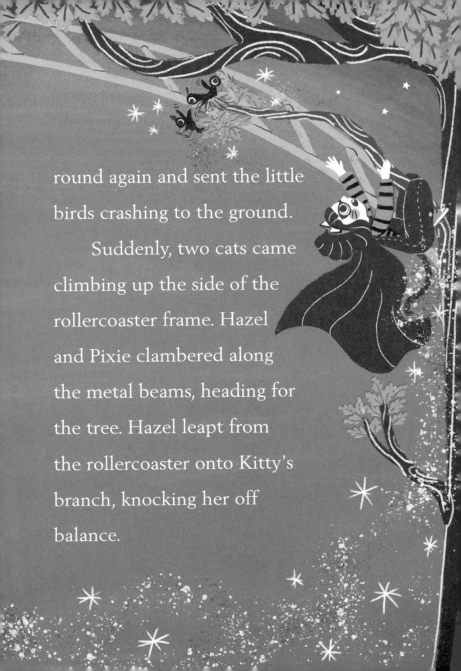

round again and sent the little birds crashing to the ground.

Suddenly, two cats came climbing up the side of the rollercoaster frame. Hazel and Pixie clambered along the metal beams, heading for the tree. Hazel leapt from the rollercoaster onto Kitty's branch, knocking her off balance.

Kitty steadied herself as the branch wobbled. 'Hey, what's going on?' she asked, but Hazel ignored her.

Pixie leapt from the rollercoaster to the branch and followed Hazel up the tree. 'Hi, Kitty. I can't stop,' she mewed. 'We're rescuing creatures in peril!'

'Pixie—wait!' called Kitty, but Pixie had already dashed away to join her friend.

Hazel grabbed the birds' nest, making it tip even further. One of the little birds slipped out and its stubby

wings fluttered in panic.
Luckily, Pixie caught the bird
and put it back into the nest
again.

'Stop that silly cheeping!' Hazel
told the birds rudely. 'I am a Cat
Superhero and I know exactly what I'm
doing.' She grabbed the side of the nest
with her mouth and began making her
way down the tree.

Kitty also began to climb again,
her eyes fixed on the little birds. When
Hazel made an extra big jump and lost

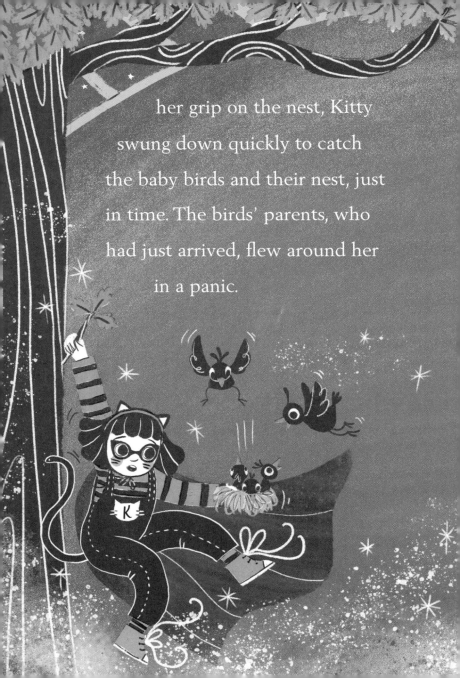

her grip on the nest, Kitty
swung down quickly to catch
the baby birds and their nest, just
in time. The birds' parents, who
had just arrived, flew around her
in a panic.

'It's all right!' Kitty told them. 'Your babies are much safer away from that rollercoaster.' She turned to find the next foothold, but Hazel snatched the nest back without even saying thank you.

Kitty followed the two cats, sighing with relief when they reached the bottom without dropping the birds. 'You have to be more careful!' she said, as Hazel dumped the nest on the ground. 'These little birds were in terrible danger . . .'

'YOU shouldn't get in the way!' interrupted Hazel. 'You could have ruined the whole mission. *I* had everything under control because *I* am a real Cat Superhero, not just a silly human pretending to be a cat.'

'That's not fair at all!' cried Kitty. Hazel twitched her whiskers and gave Kitty a cold stare.

'Pixie is MY sidekick now. She doesn't need YOU anymore! You should leave the superhero stuff to us from now on.'

Pixie glanced sideways at Kitty before turning away quickly.

Kitty felt tears prick her eyes. She hadn't expected Hazel to be so mean. Why hadn't Pixie stuck up for her? She'd thought they were friends.

'Anyway, we can't hang around here chatting to you,' Hazel went on.

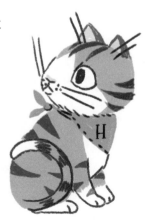

'We have important rescue work to
do. Come on, Pixie!' She marched off,
ignoring the cheeping birds in their nest
on the ground.

Pixie slunk after her.

Kitty knelt down and took the
birds' nest carefully in her hands.

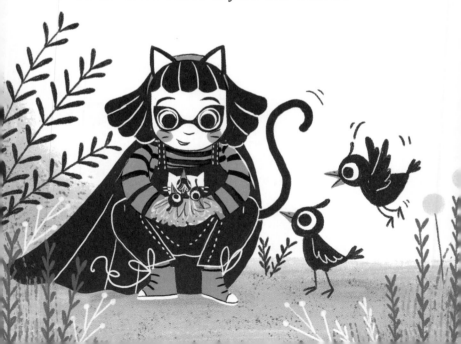

'Kitty, what happened?' Figaro came running up with Pumpkin beside him. 'We saw Hazel and Pixie at the top of the tree.'

'I think they wanted to be the ones to save the day,' said Kitty. 'Or maybe they didn't believe I'd manage the rescue by myself.'

Figaro shook his head. 'That Hazel is a menace! I don't know why Pixie thinks she's so wonderful. I didn't see her use any superpowers at all!'

Kitty looked down at the three little birds huddled together in the nest. Their parents were fussing over them worriedly. The baby birds stared back at Kitty with wide eyes. Keeping them safe was what mattered now. 'Let's find a better place to put your nest,' she said. 'I think you need a nice place to sleep.'

The largest fledgling piped up in a tiny voice, 'I'm too excited to sleep. That was my very first adventure and I think it was amazing!'

Kitty smiled and stroked his feathery head. 'I'm just glad you're OK. Shall we find a new home for you?'

'How about that hawthorn bush? I'm sure it'll be nice and quiet in there.' Pumpkin nodded to a patch of brambles away from the bright lights and the noise of the rides.

'Oh, yes please!' said the baby birds' father. 'That would be a wonderful place for our nest.'

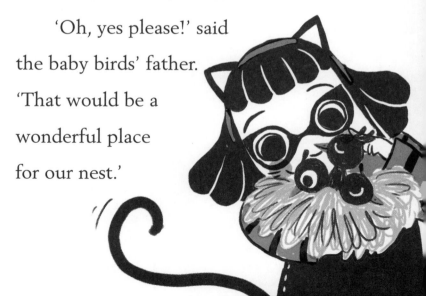

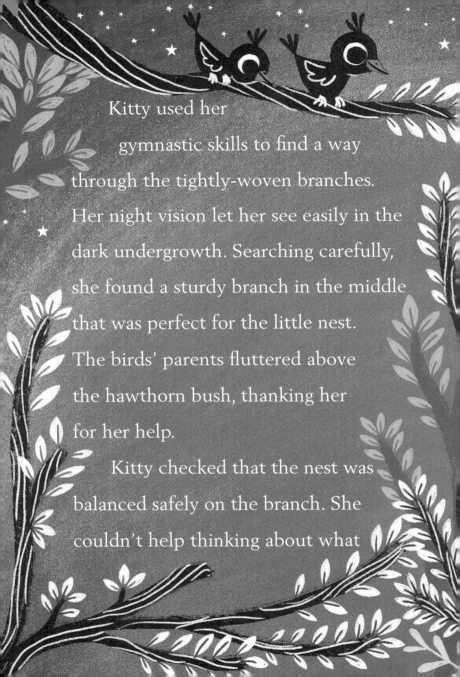

Kitty used her

gymnastic skills to find a way

through the tightly-woven branches.

Her night vision let her see easily in the

dark undergrowth. Searching carefully,

she found a sturdy branch in the middle

that was perfect for the little nest.

The birds' parents fluttered above

the hawthorn bush, thanking her

for her help.

Kitty checked that the nest was

balanced safely on the branch. She

couldn't help thinking about what

Hazel had said to her: *I am a real Cat Superhero, not just a silly human pretending to be a cat.* That wasn't fair at all. She wasn't pretending to be anything.

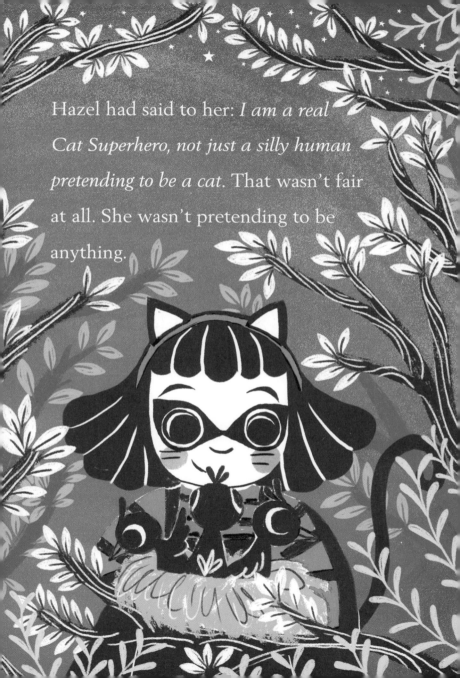

She swallowed, wondering whether Pixie or Figaro had ever thought she was trying to be a cat too.

'Can I come on another adventure with you?' asked the largest fledgling. 'Please? It was such a lot of fun!'

'I don't think that's a good idea,' Kitty replied. 'You're a bit young to be having adventures.' She turned away, still thinking about Hazel and Pixie.

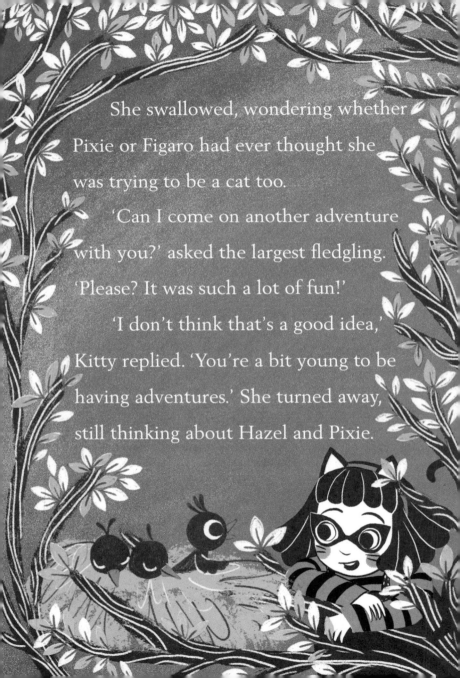

The baby bird gave a disappointed cheep before huddling down inside the nest with his brother and sister. Kitty slipped through the tangle of branches and headed back towards the flashing lights of the funfair. She met Figaro and Pumpkin and they spotted Kitty's family at the toffee apple stand.

'Is everything all right, Kitty?' asked Pumpkin.

'I was thinking about Pixie and how excited she is to have made

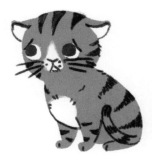

friends with Hazel.' Kitty sighed. She missed the little white cat terribly, but Pixie hadn't even stuck up for her when Hazel had said mean things.

Kitty was silent most of the way home. Her feet felt heavy and her head was pounding after the loud funfair music.

'Is something wrong?' her mum asked her quietly. 'You haven't said anything since we left the fair.'

'No, not really,' said Kitty. 'It's just . . . I thought everyone would understand that I'm just trying to help people with my superpowers.'

Her mum put an arm around her. 'Being a superhero isn't always easy. Sometimes other people won't understand what you're trying to do, but that doesn't mean you should give up. There are people and animals out there that will need your help. Remember—you're stronger than you think!'

'Thanks, Mum.' Kitty gave her a hug. Her heart felt a little lighter as

they headed home in the moonlight.
She knew she had tried to help the
birds the best she could.

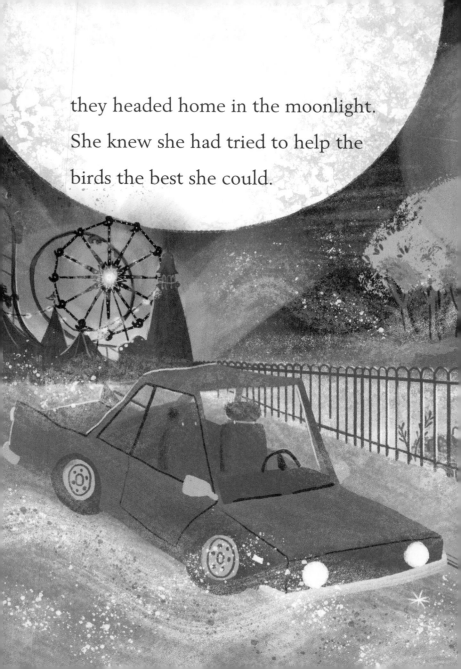

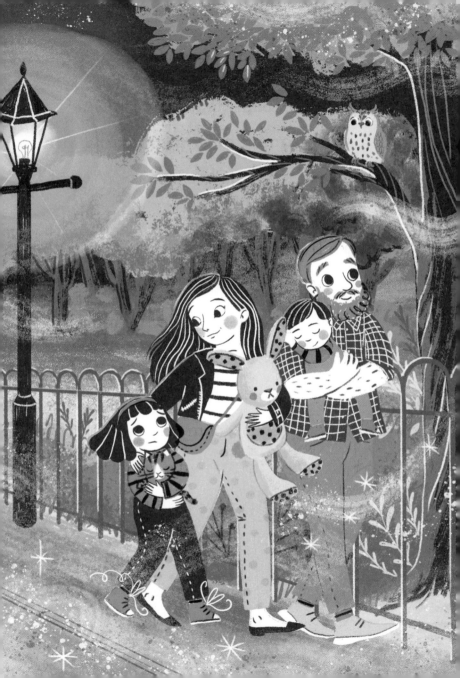

Chapter 4

That night, Kitty dreamt
that she was stuck on the Merry-Go-
Round at the fair. Pixie was there too,
eating candy floss and giggling with
Hazel. The Merry-Go-Round spun
faster and faster and made her dizzy.

Then she heard Figaro shouting her name and his voice grew louder and louder and louder.

Kitty sat up straight in bed. The wind whispered at the open window, making the curtains sway. She rubbed her eyes sleepily. She could still hear Figaro calling her. That part wasn't a dream at all!

She slipped out of bed, careful not to disturb Pumpkin, who was asleep on her pillow. Running to the window, she peered out into the darkness.

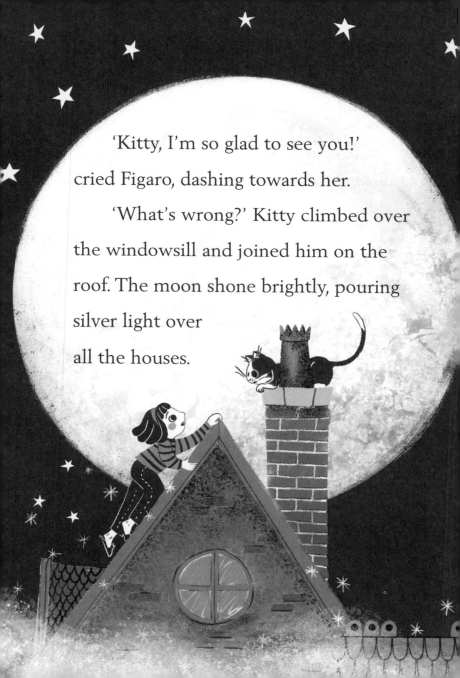

'Kitty, I'm so glad to see you!'
cried Figaro, dashing towards her.

'What's wrong?' Kitty climbed over
the windowsill and joined him on the
roof. The moon shone brightly, pouring
silver light over
all the houses.

'It's Pixie and Hazel!' puffed
Figaro, trying to catch his breath.

Kitty's eyes widened in alarm.
Figaro always liked to be dignified and
grand. She'd never seen him rush about
like this before. His black-and-white fur
was standing on end and his whiskers
were shaking.

'They've gone too far this time . . .
they're in terrible danger!' he went
on. 'We must leave for the fairground
immediately.'

Kitty dashed inside and put on her

superhero outfit. If Pixie was in trouble she would be there to help, no matter what had happened earlier that evening. Tying her black cape around her neck, she sprang back out of the window. Her superpowers tingled inside her like electricity and her heartbeat quickened.

Pumpkin had woken up and he followed her to the window. 'What's happening?' he asked.

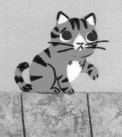

'Pixie's in trouble! We have to hurry.' Kitty gathered Pumpkin into her arms and dashed after Figaro.

The city streets below were quiet. Only the occasional hoot of an owl or the rustle of a mouse broke the silence. Kitty and Figaro raced across the rooftops. They climbed drainpipes, jumped over chimney pots, and swung around satellite dishes. At last, Kitty spotted the fairground in the distance.

Figaro leapt on to the pavement and ran down the alley that led to the fair.

The rides were still and silent, and the food stands were empty. The only thing moving was an empty crisp packet blowing across the grass.

Kitty shivered. The fair looked spooky in the dark. Then she took a deep breath. She was here to help Pixie and Hazel, she reminded herself. There was no time to be scared!

Figaro stopped at the bottom of the Big Wheel. 'I told them not to go up there!' he cried. 'If only they had listened to me.'

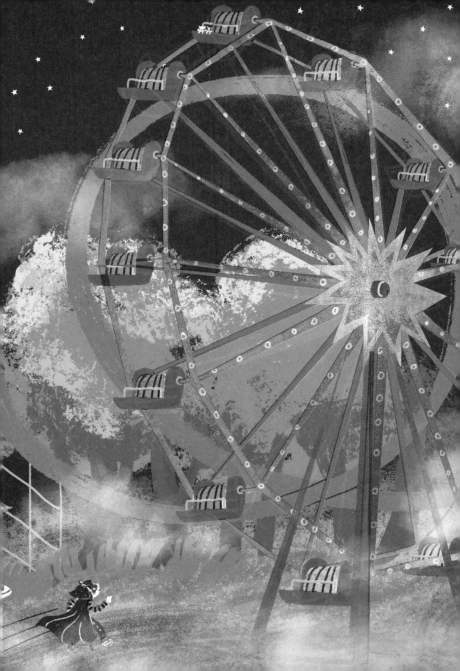

Kitty gazed at the huge Big Wheel with its round frame and crisscrossing metal beams. The moon had risen behind the ride and the shiny metal frame glinted in the pale light. Kitty spotted two tiny shapes right at the top of the wheel. Hazel was hanging from the frame by the tips of her paws. Pixie was dangling from Hazel's tail.

Kitty gulped. The ride's metal frame was made from narrow beams. They looked slippery and hard to climb. No wonder Pixie and Hazel were in such terrible trouble.

'Pixie said they'd seen a creature in danger,' Figaro told Kitty. 'And that's why they decided to go up there.'

Pumpkin gasped. 'But it's such a long way to fall!'

Kitty used her special night vision to zoom in on the frightened cats at the top of the ride.

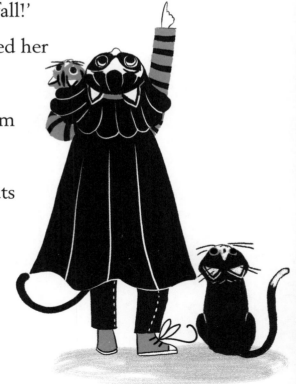

She suddenly wondered whether Hazel's tales of superpowers had been true, but there was no time to think about that now. 'Don't worry!' she told Pumpkin. 'I can reach them.'

'Be careful, Kitty!' cried Figaro.

Kitty began climbing the frame of the ride, using the crisscrossing metal beams.

'We're up here, Kitty. Please help us!' Pixie wailed from high above.

Kitty's heart raced and she climbed even faster. Rain began to fall, making

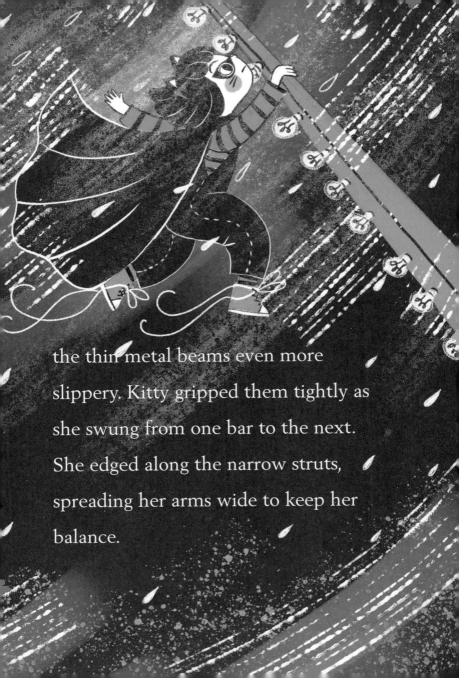

the thin metal beams even more
slippery. Kitty gripped them tightly as
she swung from one bar to the next.
She edged along the narrow struts,
spreading her arms wide to keep her
balance.

When she glanced at the ground, her heart skipped a beat. It really was a long way down. *You can do this*, she told herself. *You're a superhero in training!*

The wind grew stronger, blowing raindrops into Kitty's face. Water dripped from her black cape, but she went on climbing bravely. She was determined to reach the cats, no matter how difficult it was.

'Hurry, Kitty!' squeaked Pixie. 'I don't think I can hold on much longer.'

Kitty looked up in alarm. Pixie had

slipped down
Hazel's tail and
was holding on
with one paw.
Pumpkin and
Figaro's scared
faces gazed up
at them from the
ground far below.

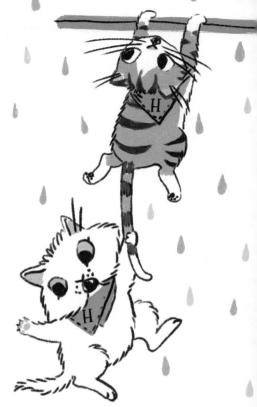

'Hold on! I'm nearly there.' Kitty
jumped on to one of the Big Wheel's
cars and went on climbing.

At last, she reached the top of the

ride. Balancing on the highest beam, she pulled Hazel up with both hands. Hazel's fur stood on end and her paws trembled as Kitty set her safely down on the beam.

Just as Kitty was about to scoop Pixie up, a torrent of rain pelted them all. Pixie let out a terrible screech, losing her grip on Hazel's tail and tumbling downwards. Quick as a whisker, Kitty hooked her feet over the metal bar and swung through the air like an acrobat.

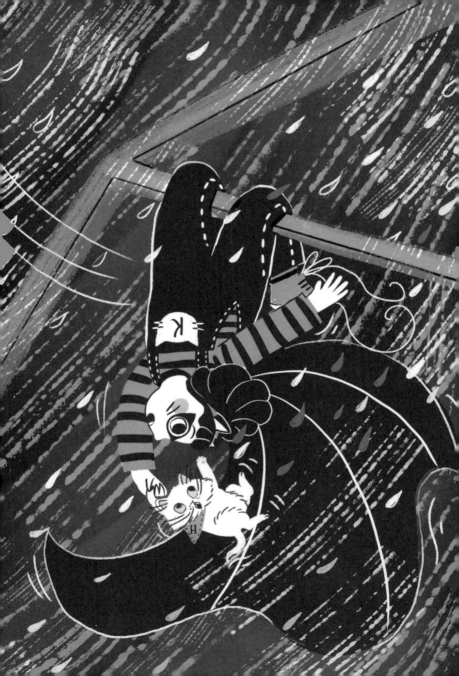

The night breeze whooshed past her. She grabbed hold of Pixie's paws and held the cat tightly as they swung together. Then she dropped Pixie neatly inside one of the cars. As she swung back to the beam, she nearly lost her balance. For a terrible moment, she stared at the ground far below. Then she grabbed the beam with one hand and pulled herself to safety.

Hazel stared at her open-mouthed, her whiskers shaking.

Kitty tried to catch her breath but her heart was racing. 'Are you all right?' she asked Hazel.

'YOWL!' cried Hazel, tears rolling down her cheeks.

Kitty lifted Hazel carefully with one arm and climbed down to the car where she'd left Pixie. The two cats huddled together on the seats while Kitty perched on the bars in front.

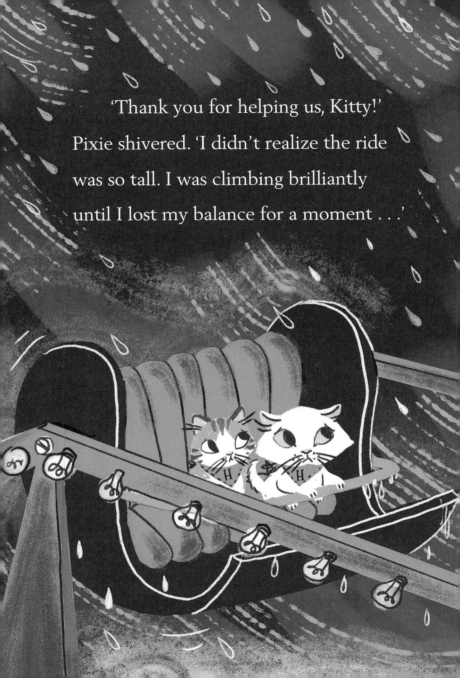

'Thank you for helping us, Kitty!'
Pixie shivered. 'I didn't realize the ride
was so tall. I was climbing brilliantly
until I lost my balance for a moment . . .'

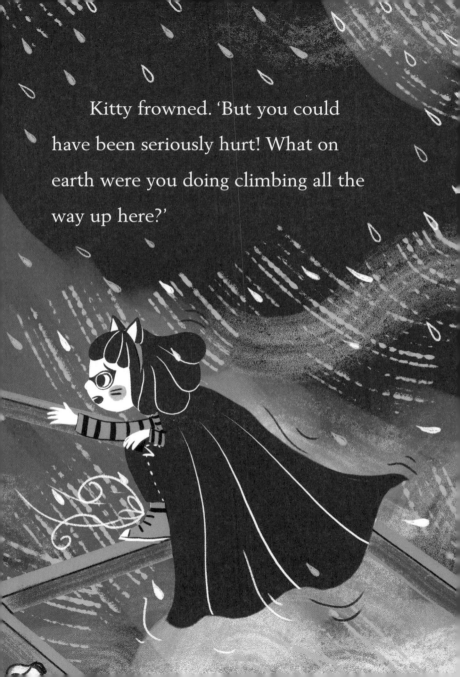

Kitty frowned. 'But you could have been seriously hurt! What on earth were you doing climbing all the way up here?'

Chapter

5

Hazel and Pixie sat hunched
in the car at the top of the Big Wheel.
Hazel's whiskers were still shaking.

'You're safe now,' Kitty said more
gently. 'But tell me why you came
up here. Figaro said there was an

animal in danger.'

'We saw a baby bird stuck at the top and we climbed up to save him . . .' Hazel mumbled. 'But then we slipped and got into trouble.'

'Where did you see the bird?' asked Kitty, alarmed.

'On one of those cars.' Pixie pointed upwards. 'But I can't see him anymore.'

Kitty peered at the cars hanging overhead. The wind blew strongly, making them rock. 'Wait for me here!'

she told the cats. Then she sprang for the nearest beam and ran along the frame of the ride. She searched the first car but found nothing. Climbing to the next one, she heard a tiny chirping sound.

'Hello,' she called. 'My name's Kitty. Are you all right?'

'Oh dear!' cheeped a small voice. 'How will I ever get down?'

'I'll help you! Please don't worry.' Kitty hunted all around and found the baby bird clinging to the back of the car.

His feathers were ruffled and his eyes were wide with fright. Kitty scooped him up and settled him on her shoulder.

'Oh, thank you!' he squeaked, clinging to her with his stubby wings.

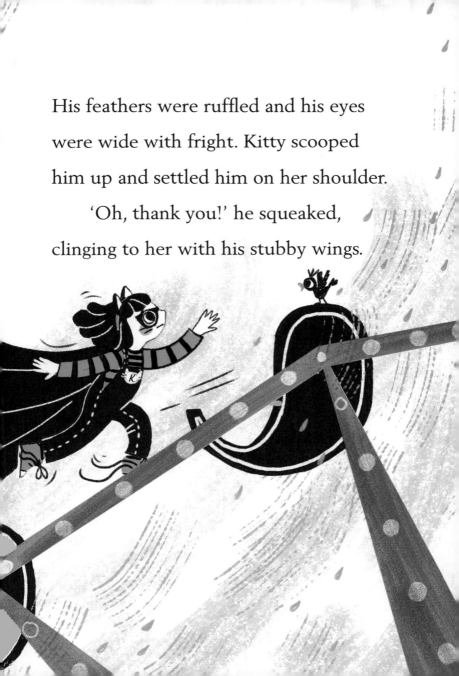

'That's all right!' Kitty looked more closely. She was sure she recognized the little bird. 'Aren't you one of the birds from the nest beside the rollercoaster? Why are you all the way up here?'

The bird snuggled against Kitty's neck. 'I just wanted to prove that I'm old enough to have an adventure. I thought it would be exciting, but it's horrible and scary and I want to go home!'

'But how did you get

here?' asked Kitty. 'It's a very long way from your nest.'

'I hid in one of the cars when no one was looking,' the baby bird said. 'Then the ride stopped and everyone went home. That's when I knew I was stuck because I haven't learnt how to fly yet. I tried to hop back down but I just couldn't!'

Kitty's heart sank. She remembered that the little bird had wanted an adventure and she had said he was too young. If she had taken more time to talk to him he might never have put himself in danger. She had been upset after Hazel called her *a silly human* and that had pushed everything else out of her head.

'I know I said you were too young for adventures but that was unfair of me,' she told the baby bird. 'Once you've learnt to fly we could go on an adventure together. Would you like that?'

'Yes please! I'd love that,' the bird said eagerly.

'Then I promise you that's what

we'll do!' Kitty smiled at the bird and he flapped his wings happily.

Kitty checked he was perched safely on her shoulder before climbing back to Pixie and Hazel. The wind blew in strong gusts, making the Big Wheel cars rock to and fro.

'We'd better climb down quickly,' Kitty told the cats. 'It's not safe to stay up here in such a strong wind.'

'I can't!' Hazel's voice wobbled. 'I'm worried that I'll slip again.'

'I'll help you. Climb on to my arm.'

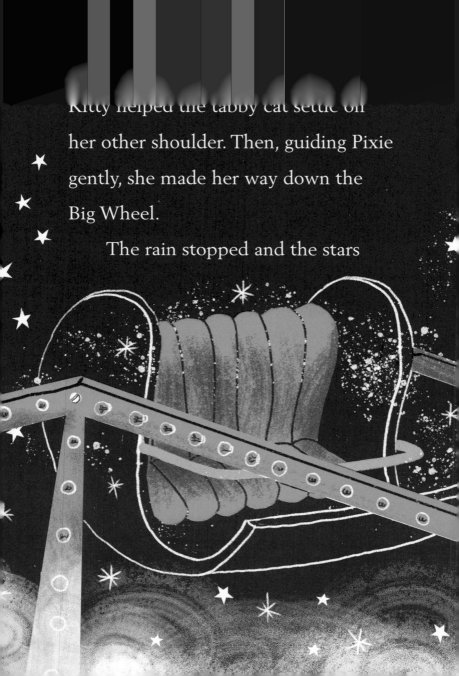

Kitty helped the tabby cat settle on her other shoulder. Then, guiding Pixie gently, she made her way down the Big Wheel.

The rain stopped and the stars

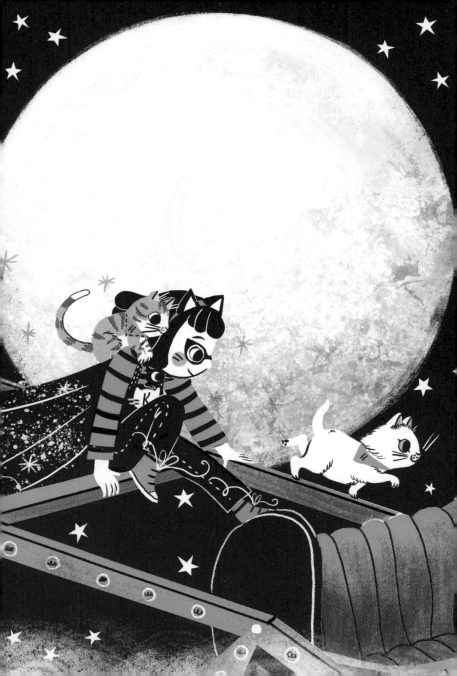

appeared again, twinkling like diamonds in the dark sky. Kitty clambered down slowly, careful not to slip on the wet beams. At last she leapt gracefully from the Big Wheel to the ground.

'Hurrah, you're all safe!' Pumpkin jumped around and waved his stripy tail.

'Thank goodness!' Figaro gave a dramatic sigh.

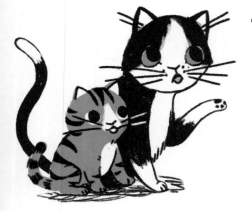

'I was afraid that something truly terrible would

happen. All the time you were up there I could hardly look!'

Kitty had expected Pixie to start chattering about everything they'd done, but instead the little white cat burst into tears. 'I'm really sorry, Kitty,' she sobbed. 'I didn't mean to cause so much trouble. I thought Hazel was a superhero in training just like you and that everything would be all right!'

Figaro shook his head. 'I KNEW the superhero thing couldn't be real.'

Hazel stared down at her paws.

'I just liked pretending,' she muttered. 'And I really *was* worried about the baby bird.'

'You shouldn't have done it!' snapped Figaro. 'I had to run all the way to Kitty's house when you got yourselves stuck. I nearly grazed my paw on a chimney pot.'

'It's all right, Figaro.' Kitty shushed him.

Tears were dripping down Pixie's cheeks. Hazel stared at the ground, her tail drooping.

'I think you made some mistakes,' said Kitty. 'But you were also very brave. Not many cats would have had the courage to climb all the way up the Big Wheel.'

Pixie sniffed and wiped her cheek with her paw.

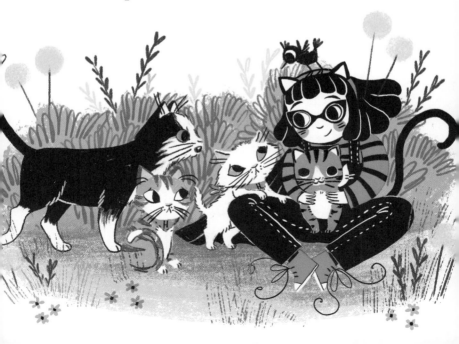

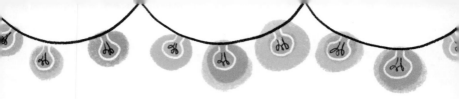

Kitty tried to think of what her mum would say. 'I know you wanted to be like superheroes. But I think being a superhero is about more than being brave. It's about being kind too and looking for the best in others—animals and humans.' She smiled at the baby bird still perched on her shoulder. 'You can't help others if you can't be kind.'

Hazel nodded. 'I'm sorry, Kitty. I shouldn't have been so unfair to you. Do you think . . . um . . . that we could be friends?'

'Of course we can!' Kitty smiled.

'I'm sorry too!' Pixie perked up
a little. 'I missed being part of the cat
crew and meeting up at your house,
Kitty. Do you think we could go back
there now all together?'

'I think that's the best
idea in the world!'
said Kitty.

Chapter
6

Kitty took the baby bird
back to his nest in the bushes. The
bird's parents had returned after
hunting for grubs. They thanked Kitty
for looking after their baby again, and
snuggled down together for the night.

Pixie led the way out of the dark fairground. Kitty walked alongside Hazel, who cast shy glances up at her. They climbed the drainpipe at the end of the alley and scampered along the rooftops back to Kitty's house. Hazel followed Kitty, trying to copy the way she jumped and ran.

The clouds drifted away and the moon shone even brighter than before. The roofs glistened with thousands of raindrops and each puddle on the pavement reflected a tiny pale moon.

Kitty smiled widely as they reached the flat roof above her bedroom. She was so happy to have her friends together again. She somersaulted over the chimney pot, her long cape flying out around her.

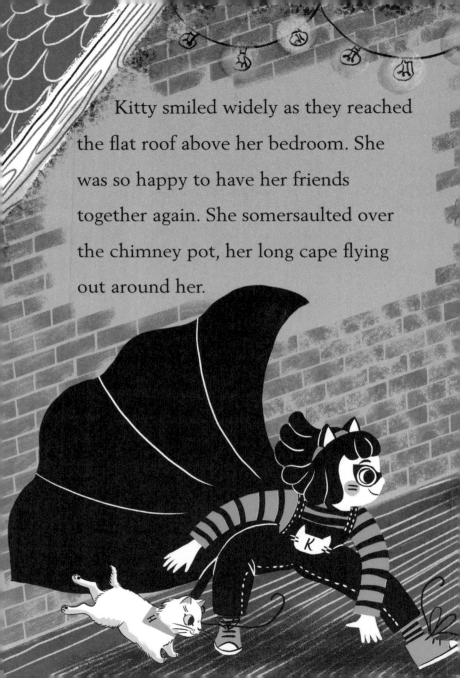

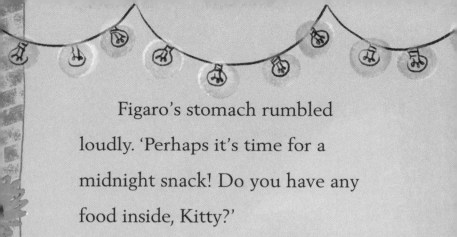

Figaro's stomach rumbled
loudly. 'Perhaps it's time for a
midnight snack! Do you have any
food inside, Kitty?'

'My Dad bought some fresh
mackerel from the fishmongers
today,' Kitty told him. 'I'll bring
everything outside and we can have
a proper midnight feast.'

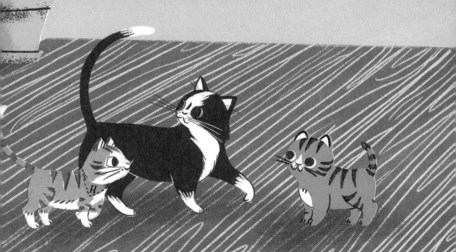

'I'll help you, Kitty!' meowed Pumpkin.

Kitty and Pumpkin climbed inside and gathered everything into a picnic basket. There were orange plates and bowls, and a picnic rug covered in a paw pattern. Kitty added some homemade chocolate chip cookies to the basket and a bottle of milk.

Returning to the rooftop, she found Hazel listening to Figaro as he explained how important it was to groom her tail and whiskers correctly.

'Always start at the root of your
fur and then groom outwards with
one smooth movement!' he said,
demonstrating with a grand flourish.

Pixie bounced up and down when
she saw the picnic basket. 'Ooh, thanks
Kitty! Let me help you with the rug.'

They laid the rug on the flat
rooftop and Kitty shared out the pieces
of mackerel. Pixie also took a cookie as
she loved anything with chocolate.

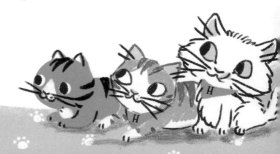

Hazel took a nibble of her fish.

Then she gave a shy cough.

'Um . . . Kitty? It must be amazing to be a superhero. I've never seen anyone climb and balance like you can. I would love to be just like you!'

'Kitty is the best!' said Pumpkin. 'We've had so many adventures together.'

Hazel twitched her whiskers eagerly. 'I'd like to hear about them. That's if you don't mind!'

'All right! Let me think . . .' Kitty brushed the cookie crumbs from her hands. 'I know! There was once a precious Golden Tiger statue that was stolen from the museum. Its eyes were made of real emeralds and it had a special secret . . .'

Hazel's eyes grew wider as Kitty told her all about the thief that stole the tiger statue, and how she got it back. Figaro added a few details to the story here and there.

The moon smiled down at the

rooftop and the stars twinkled. Kitty
looked at the eager faces of the cats and
she felt a warm glow spread inside her.
It was wonderful to jump and climb
and turn somersaults, but having good
friends was really special too.

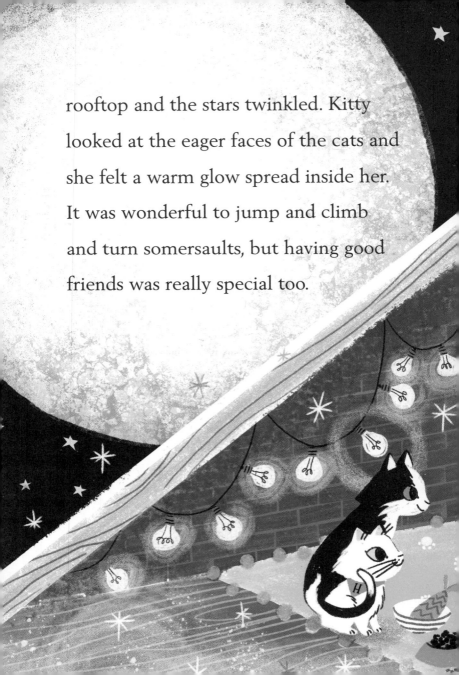

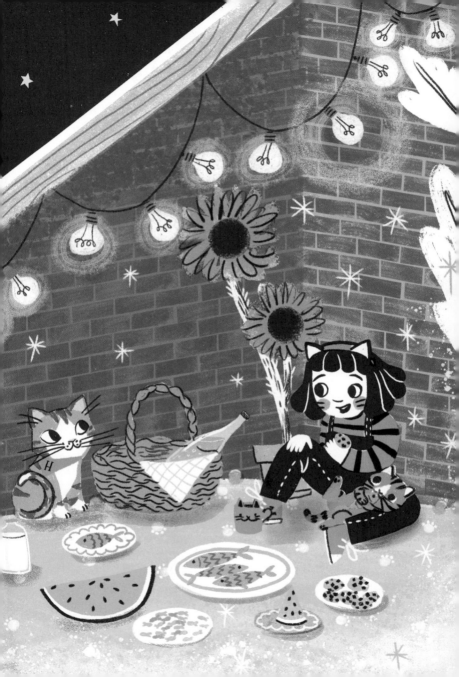

Super Facts About Cats

Super Speed

Have you ever seen a cat make a quick escape from a dog? If so, you'll know that they can move *really* fast—up to 30mph!

Super Hearing

Cats have an incredible sense of hearing and can swivel their large ears to pinpoint even the tiniest of sounds.

Super Reflexes

Have you ever heard the saying 'cats always land on their feet'? People say this because cats have amazing reflexes. If a cat is falling, they can sense quickly how to move their bodies into the right position to land safely.

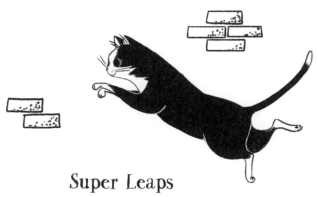

Super Leaps

A cat can jump over eight feet high
in a single leap; this is due to its powerful
back leg muscles.

Super Vision

Cats have amazing night-time vision. Their
incredible ability to see in low light allows them
to hunt for prey when it's dark outside.

Super Smell

Cats have a very powerful sense of smell,
14 times stronger than a human's. Did you know
that the pattern of ridges on each cat's nose
is as unique as a human's fingerprint?

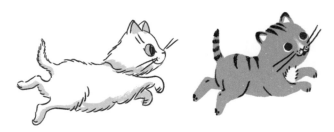

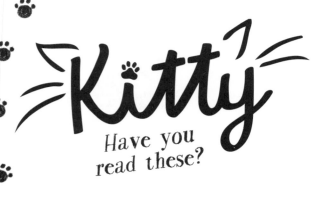

Kitty

Have you read these?

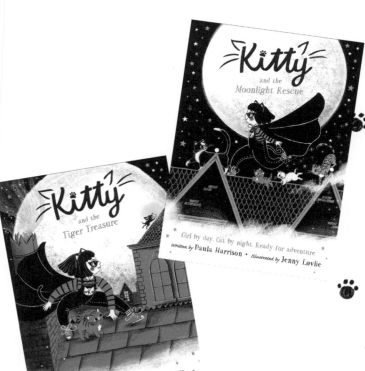

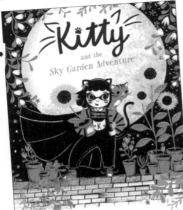

Kitty
and the
Sky Garden Adventure

✻ Girl by day. Cat by night. Ready for adventure. *✻*
Written by **Paula Harrison** • *Illustrated by* **Jenny Løvlie**

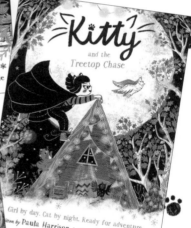

Kitty
and the
Treetop Chase

Girl by day. Cat by night. Ready for adventure.
Written by **Paula Harrison** • *Illustrated by* **Jenny Løvlie**

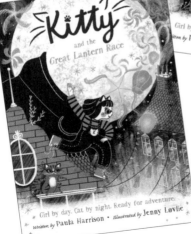

Kitty
and the
Great Lantern Race

Girl by day. Cat by night. Ready for adventure.
✻ *Written by* **Paula Harrison** • *Illustrated by* **Jenny Løvlie** *✻*

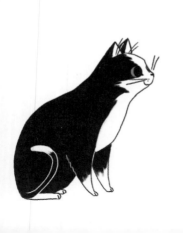

About the author

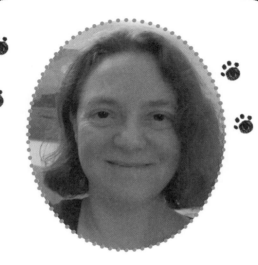

Paula Harrison

Before launching a successful writing career,
Paula was a Primary school teacher. Her years teaching
taught her what children like in stories and how
they respond to humour and suspense. She went on
to put her experience to good use, writing many
successful stories for young readers.

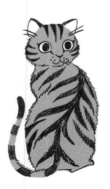

About the illustrator

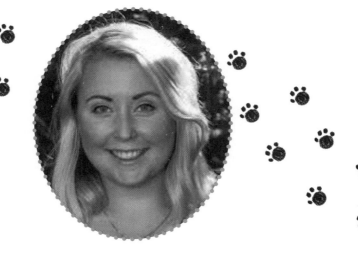

Jenny Løvlie

Jenny is a Norwegian illustrator, designer,
creative, foodie, and bird enthusiast. She is fascinated
by the strong bond between humans and animals and
loves using bold colours and shapes in her work.

Love Kitty?
Why not try these too . . .

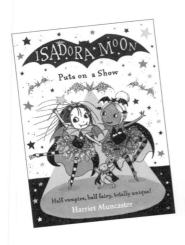

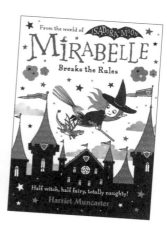

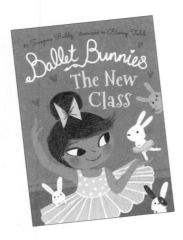

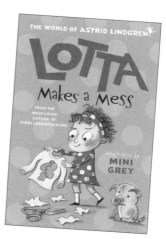